"Louisa Maccan-Graves is rapidly becoming the Martha Stewart of beauty and I predict her book will soon become the 'bible of beauty' for all appearance-conscious women (and many men as well). One good look at this remarkable woman's skin, face, neck and hands, and you'll gladly shell out the price of this book to learn her secrets. It contains a wealth of useful and practical information. It is extremely well-organized and is written in a no-nonsense, easy-to-follow style."
F. A. Cord, MD

"...As the Chairman of Integrative Medicine and Anti-Aging Conferences, I believe that Louisa has put something together here of significant practical value. Along with four other physicians, I also recommend *"Hollywood Beauty Secrets: Remedies to the Rescue"* as a "must read" for all women who care about their health and appearance. May I add that my wife, Lori uses and recommends the effective anti-aging tips in Louisa's book."
L. Stephen Coles, M.D.

"*Hollywood Beauty Secrets: Remedies to the Rescue* is a concise insight to the personal care world of a career professional model. Louisa's book takes you through core issues of personal appearance, wellness, anti-aging skin care and her secrets to access affordable and effective products and rejuvenating therapies. Everyone, men included, may benefit with her secrets to success! Hollywood Beauty Secrets is an important work for all aesthetic medicine and surgery professionals to recommend for their clients."
R. S. Jennings, MD

"A great book, full of insightful tips. Not surprising, from a woman who not only looks years younger than her age, but maintains her own health so carefully and well."
C. Ott, MD

"Being a make-up artist in the film industry, I try hundreds of products, but nothing has hydrated and smoothed my skin the moisturizer and the Microdermabrasion Scrub Louisa suggest in her book. Within two days of using them, I saw immediate results!! My skin felt smooth, moist, firm and lines around my eyes softened. Louisa has certainly uncovered amazing skin care products that work far better than any expensive or hyped product on the market."
Linda V., Hollywood Make-up Artist

"I thoroughly enjoyed and highly recommend Louisa's book, Hollywood Beauty Secrets: Remedies to the Rescue." I believe every woman will find this complete beauty guide is loaded with insightful and invaluable beauty remedies. Everything is doable, affordable and really works!"
Sue S., Medical Aesthetician

"Louisa is considered an anomaly in fiercely competitive Hollywood where most women will never reveal their beauty secrets."
Nicole M., Reporter

"On a beauty budget? In the days of $250 DNA face creams and expensive plastic surgery, wrinkle injections, and chemical peels, how refreshing it is to find a book which outlines inexpensive beauty buys to remedy everything from battling blemishes, weight loss, plumping lips, and rejuvenating facial and body skin. Hollywood Beauty Secrets - Remedies to the

Rescue is a godsend for those looking for low budget ways to look and feel great. This is a refreshing and interesting read, worthwhile to anyone who is watching their pennies. Let's face it - being beautiful shouldn't have to cost an arm and a leg and Louisa shows us the way."
Anne G.

"I just had to drop you a note .... I am having so much fun with your book, "Hollywood Beauty Secrets: Remedies to the Rescue." I have shared it with my co-workers and it has gone out to lunch with more people than I have! I've decided to buy two more copies of the book to share with my friends. Thanks Louisa, your booked is filled with fantastic health and beauty advice that really works!"
Tricia B.

"I know Louisa through my work in the commercial film industry, where we spend long hours on our feet, days on end. I love her easy, thirty-minute pedicure! My feet have never been so happy, or so pretty! All of Louisa's advice is directed to busy women like me who need simple, economical, practical ways to take care of our bodies."
Carol C.

"I so enjoyed reading Louisa's book, "Hollywood Beauty Secrets: Remedies to the Rescue." It's a rich treasure chest of remedies and ideas to enable any woman to target problem spots and overcome them. Louisa doesn't resort to fluff to fill in space and sell more books but fills every page with substantial, quality suggestions as to how to attend to problem spots utilizing such readily available ingredients as milk, baking soda and coffee grounds. I found myself continually saying, "wow - I didn't know that!" I now use many of Louisa's

recommendations and feel better than ever! In a town filled with fierce competition and desire for personal gain, it is tempting for beautiful women to keep beauty secrets to themselves. It is so refreshing to read a book from an author that cares enough to share her secrets so that every woman has the opportunity to be her very best."
Jennifer M.

"I enjoyed Hollywood Beauty Secrets: Remedies to the Rescue" so much! In fact, I've read through it twice and devoured so much information. I also want to order more books for my friends!"
Pat B.

"Hollywood Beauty Secrets: Remedies to the Rescue is an amazing compilation of practical, tried and true remedies for beauty concerns most women face at some point in their lives. Let Louisa's track record speak for itself, and let her remedies change your life forever."
Maria T.D.

"There is absolutely no other book on the market like "Hollywood Beauty Secrets: Remedies to the Rescue." It is filled with doable, invaluable beauty advice that every woman on the planet has been looking for. Louisa's extensive modeling career certainly indicates that she must be doing something right!"
Trudy N.

"Your book has provided me with a sensible, affordable 'user-friendly' guide to help keep my skin, hair and nails in perfect condition. I tell everyone about your book. It's a must read!"
Marlene H.

"I am exposed to the sun quite regularly which concerned me. I learned from Louisa's book that only a few sunscreens contain effective UV protection. I e-mailed the effective ingredients she specified to look for on sunscreen labels to all my friends and they in turn e-mailed their friends. Louisa helped a lot of people who were misinformed about sun protection."
Lee A.

"Ok, I have a story about the author, Louisa Maccan-Graves. About 6 months ago I was in my doctor's waiting room when he approached me and asked if I would mind speaking about my treatments to a woman that was writing a book on beauty solutions. I agreed to talk to her for 2 reasons: I felt that if any woman that shared my problem of unsightly cellulite could get help from my experience, then I wanted to be a part of that and also because the woman (Louisa) seemed very personable. She was very thorough in her questioning in the office and called me later that day to ask me even more Q's. I allowed her access to my before photos so she could be certain I was not imagining my progress. She has kept a steady vigilance of following up with me to hear if my improvements were continuing and holding. A few times I took advantage of her calls and asked about unrelated problems I was having, she gave me several remedies that I am still using today and they were inexpensive and they really work. So I rated her book upon a first hand trust factor, I know she does her homework, I know she asks the hard questions and demands proof and I know she has a great deal of information on many beauty solutions in that pretty head of hers."
Barbara A.

3rd Edition
Published by
Bella Publications
Copyright (c) 2003, 2004 by Louisa Maccan-Graves
ISBN # 0-9760913-0-5
Library of Congress Catalog Card Number: 2003113218

Editing by: Jennifer Matney, Marlene Harryman and Maria DeAngelus.
Formatting: Marcel Esser & Erika Wheeler
Cover Design: Hunter Business Forms, Inc. Print & Promotions, Canada
Manufactured in the United States of America

Hollywood
Beauty Secrets:
Remedies to the Rescue

by
Louisa Maccan-Graves

Bella Publications

Contents

Part One:
Making Time For You

Part Two:
Facial Care

Part Three:
Special Skin Needs

Part Four:
Eye Care

Part Five:
Lip & Oral Care

Part Six:
Nail, Hand & Foot Care

Part Seven:
Leg & Body Care

Part Eight:
Boost Your Metabolism

Part Nine:
PMS & Balancing Hormones

Part Ten:
Hair Care

11

Part Eleven:
Medicine Cabinet

Part Twelve:
Anti-Aging Alternatives

13

Acknowledgments

This book is dedicated to the love of my life, my husband John Graves! I could have never completed this project without your love, support and patience. I would also like to thank my wonderful parents, sisters, brother and relatives for their support and encouragement. A special thanks to Angela Tisiot at Hunter Business forms for the cover design and thanks to Marcel Esser and Erika Wheeler for your patience formatting my book. Special thanks to editors and proofreaders, Dr. F. Coard, Jennifer Matney, Marlene Harryman, Caren Larkey-Lewis and Maria DeAngelus. Thanks to both my personal and professional friends Jennifer, Robin, Dru, Isabelle, Vickie, Caren, Marlene, Summer, Lori, Ellen, Grace, Lisa, Pat, Sue, Annie, Suzanne, and Nicol for cheering me on. A great big, special thanks goes out to each and every contributor who shared their expertise, testimonials and beauty secrets with me over the past 20-something years. There are so many contributors, it would be difficult to list everyone and would require more space than is available. In general, the list includes dermatologists, physicians, surgeons, anti-aging experts, researchers, pharmacologists, laser specialists, medical specialists, medical aestheticians, nutritionists, manicurists, make-up artists, hair stylists, trainers, fellow models, actresses, beauty experts and private individuals. Thanks to photographers Dutch Myers (cover photo) and Carlo Bistolfi (insert photos).

Disclaimer and Important Note to the Reader

The intent of this book is to share beauty secrets. This is not a medical reference book and is not a substitution for diagnosis or treatment by a physician or health care provider. The information and advice herein is without guarantee on the part of the author, publisher or distributor and is not in any way meant to provide medical advice. Before attempting the information contained herein, CONSULT A PHYSICIAN or qualified health professional. If you are pregnant, plan to become pregnant, are breast-feeding or have problem skin or health concerns, check with your physician or dermatologist before attempting any information contained herein. The author, publisher and distributor disclaim all liability and responsibility for injury or adverse effects that may result in connection with the use of the beauty recipes, information, advice, exercises, product suggestions, doctor referrals, facilities, procedures or therapies contained herein. Consequences from use of the information contained within this book is at the reader's sole discretion and risk. It is the reader's responsibility to research supplements, side effects, procedures, doctor credentials or facilities listed within this book. Do not use recipes or products containing ingredients that you are allergic to. Should you develop an irritation or adverse reaction when utilizing any product or recipe, discontinue use immediately, remove the product with water and consult a dermatologist or physician. For medical or skin care advice, consult your physician or dermatologist.Check with your health care provider before using the slimming recipes, exercises or supplements suggested throughout the book.

Preface

Expensive doesn't always mean better! You will discover that you don't have to spend a fortune on beauty products or undergo invasive surgery to achieve rejuvenated skin, shiny hair, strong nails, smooth lips, diminish deep wrinkles, acne scars, fine lines, puffy eyes, dark circles, stretch marks, spider veins, broken capillaries, cellulite, reduce body fat and much more.

We all want to be our best. I want to share the effective, non-invasive beauty secrets that I have discovered while working as a top commercial model in Hollywood. In this book I share my own professional and personal beauty tips as well as those of dozens of Hollywood professionals and sources including dermatologists, physicians, surgeons, laser specialists, medical specialists, scientists, medical aestheticians, nutritionists, manicurists, make-up artists, hair stylists, trainers, models, actresses and private individuals. Also noted are effective products in the "Best Beauty Buys" lists that follow each remedy. Many products are reasonably priced and some can be found at most drug, health food, beauty supply or chain stores unless otherwise noted. Exceptional anti-aging therapies and beauty products noted can be found at Louisa's website. Louisa is not the manufacturer of products listed, nor was she paid to endorse products when writing this book.

NOTE: The author and contributors have not tried every product on the market and are not suggesting that other products are less effective. They are simply reporting affordable products that they feel are effective, use personally, or use in their areas of expertise.

In the Anti-Aging Alternatives section, you will find additional information about cutting-edge procedures that address specific concerns, including severe cellulite, sun damage, rosacea, port wine stains, stretch marks, et cetera. These procedures are performed by dermatologists at laser facilities and rejuvenation centers in most cities across the United States. Web sites or phone numbers have been listed where you can locate some of these services, or visit the website www.aboutskinsurgery.org. Seek the advice of your dermatologist to direct you to a facility that performs these procedures. Prices for procedures will vary from city to city. I have listed facilities in major U.S. cities, that provide treatments and services indicated. NOTE: All doctors listed are believed to be board certified medical doctors, however to be certain, it is your responsibility to research the credentials of doctors and facilities before any procedure as the author, distributor and publisher disclaim any and all liability.

About The Author

Canadian-born author **Louisa Maccan-Graves** has been a top commercial model for over 20 years, 14 of which have been in Hollywood. You may not know her name, but you have most likely seen her face, hands, lips, teeth, back, stomach, legs or bellybutton in catalogs, T.V. shows, movies and movie posters, brochures, packaging, billboards, magazines, in-store posters, infomercials, hundreds of print ads, and in more than 1000 television commercials. Louisa's face and/or body parts have graced ads and commercials for such clients as: Avon, Playtex Bra, Revlon, Dove, Cutex, L'Oreal, Clairol, Lubriderm, Almay Cosmetics, DeBeers, Mary Kaye Cosmetics, Neutrogena, Sally Hansen, Cole of California, Adidas, Sergio Valente Jeans, Tostitos, Kraft, Sears, Proctor and Gamble, TV Guide, Coke, Diet Pepsi, Dannon, Fancy Feast,Teleflora, HSN, Nail Pro, Nails Magazine, and numerous department store and jewelry catalogs, to name a few.

Louisa is best known as the top hands and/or parts model of hundreds of Hollywood actresses including: Cindy Crawford, Milla Jovovich, Sela Ward, Debra Messing, Kirsty Ally, Elaine Erwin Mellencamp, Heather Locklear, Kristen Johnson, Alyssa Milano, Patricia Heaton, Sigourney Weaver, Lauren Hutton, Victoria Jackson, Swoozie Kurtz, Cindy Taylor, Marriette Hartley, Loni Anderson, Sara O'Hare, Paulina Poriskova, Emma Samms, Madge and Caryl & Marilyn. Louisa's even poked the Pillsbury dough boy a few times!

You may have seen Louisa on television talk shows such as Tom Snyder and Talk Soup, on L.A.'s KCAL News and she recently

19

taped a segment for Emmy-Award Winning Soaptalk. You've likely heard Louisa on dozens of radio stations in Canada and the U.S. including The Wave, Kool FM and Kiss FM stations. She's featured weekly on "Louisa's Beauty Tips of the Week." Louisa is currently finishing her next book, "Hollywood Beauty Secrets: Intelligent, Affordable Anti-Aging" and she has also been a contributing writer to two local Los Angeles newspapers.

Louisa has utilized much of the information in this book throughout her 20-plus year career as a top commercial model. Included are her personal beauty secrets as well as recipes and remedies collected from dozens of beauty sources. You'll learn affordable, no-nonsense Hollywood Beauty Secrets that can help repair wrinkles, fine lines, fade pigmentation spots, relieve blemishes, acne scars, puffy eyes, dark circles, rosacea, strengthen nails, tighten skin, stimulate collagen, achieve lustrous hair, prevent falling hair, smooth stretch marks, diminish cellulite, spider veins and broken capillaries, whiten teeth, smooth cracked lips and heels, rejuvenate and brighten your complexion, enhance your mood naturally, even reverse aging using affordable products and anti-aging therapies. The no-nonsense skin care and beauty recipes listed can be done in just minutes using one or two simple household ingredients.

Louisa's methods are tried and true. Producers and directors often mistake her for at least 12 or more years younger than she is. And they consider her the best in her field as a hands and parts model in youth-oriented Hollywood. She has not had a face lift, eye lift, chemical peels, liposuction, collagen injections or invasive laser procedures. Louisa's secrets to youthful skin and a trim body are accessible, easy and no-nonsense. She has written this book for women of all ages and budgets. Every woman wants to be her best and Louisa shows you the way, affordably, safely and effectively. NOTE: Please read "Disclaimer and Important Note to the Reader" before reading on.

Foreword

Ms. Louisa Maccan-Graves, a well-known hands and body-parts model in Hollywood, has created a rich compendium of beauty tips and anti-aging secrets in one compact book for women of all ages. She informs the reader that there are many new alternative anti-aging choices available to them. Louisa offers effective anti-aging recipes and products for facial and body care, nails, hands, feet, and hair care. The book also covers insightful rejuvenating nutritional and sensible slimming information to help you lose weight. Many of the products Louisa suggests throughout the book are reasonably priced so that the budget-conscious user can shop efficiently. As the Chairman of Integrative Medicine and Anti-Aging Conferences, I believe that Louisa has put something together here of significant practical value. Along with four other physicians, I also recommend "Hollywood Beauty Secrets: Remedies to the Rescue" as a must read for all women who care about their health and appearance. May I add that my wife Lori, also uses and recommends the effective, anti-aging tips in Louisa's book.

L. Stephen Coles, M.D., Ph.D., Co-Founder of the Los Angeles Gerontology Research Group (http://www.grg.org) and Stem-Cell Researcher with the Department of Surgery in the UCLA David Geffen School of Medicine and General Chairman of the Program Committee for the Integrative Medicine and Anti-Aging Conferences (http://www.antiagingconference.com)

Introduction

Hollywood Beauty Secrets:
Remedies To The Rescue

This book was written for women of all ages. The remedies listed address the head to toe beauty concerns of all women. Men will also benefit from reading this book. It's a quick reference guide to solving skin, hair, nail and body care concerns affordably.

After each remedy, look for affordable products in the Best Beauty Buys lists. If you develop an irritation or adverse reaction, discontinue use immediately. If you have health concerns, problem skin, are pregnant, breast feeding or plan to become pregnant, consult your dermatologist or physician before attempting the information or using the recipes or products herein. NOTE: Some products may cause side effects. Best Beauty Buys products are available at most drug, health food, chain, or beauty supply stores unless otherwise noted. Harder to find items are available at www.hollywoodbeautysecrets.com. Visit the website frequently to find affordable cutting edge, anti-aging skin care products and rejuvenating therapies. NOTE: Please read the "Disclaimer and Important Note to the Reader" before you begin.

You're Number One!

As busy career women, wives or mothers we have so many responsibilities that we often don't take time for ourselves. Keep in mind that it's your responsibility to take care of your inner and outer self. In fact, when you take care of your needs first, you'll be much better equipped to give to others lovingly and without resentment.

It's never too late to make changes especially if you're currently taking on too many responsibilities. Taking on too much, creates stress that can affect both your mental and physical health, your work and your relationship with your family or partner. You may find yourself becoming impatient, upset or complaining. And you "fly off the handle" over the smallest things. Your children spend more time at their friends homes and your partner retreats to the TV, which creates even more tension. Everyone feels the tension. Your peers at work feel it, and the bottom line is — you feel it too.

Stress can take its toll on your entire body. It effects your complexion, it may be the cause of thinning or falling hair or even weight gain. Stress releases a hormone called cortisol which can contribute to weight gain in the midriff, hips and thighs. A quick solution to reducing stress and cortisol production is exercise. A simple brisk walk can help block the production of cortisol and also helps you release more endorphins which can create a "feel good" effect. Don't have time to take a walk before or after work? Find a co-worker to walk with during your lunch break. Talking while walking not only burns more calories, it helps reduce your stress levels and you'll even shed a few extra pounds.

Spending time with friends can also help reduce stress and help you live longer. A scientific study at UCLA revealed that sharing stressful events with a trusting friend or co-worker can help lower blood pressure, reduce heart disease, help you live a healthier, longer life and even help you lose a few pounds. Sharing your concerns with a friend, is not only good for your health and longevity, but can help release oxytocin, a hormone which creates a calming feeling and diminishes stress. The next time you're stressed at work or are overwhelmed with housework or errands, give your friend a call or better yet, go take a walk together.

In order to squeeze in your exercise, you have to make some changes. Ladies, it's time to do some delegating! Doing laundry, errands, house work, cooking and shopping for groceries are necessary tasks that everyone needs to learn – partners, husbands and teenagers included. Helping with housework never hurt anyone. In fact, when you teach your children these responsibilities they will be better equipped for college and they'll become more considerate partners or spouses. Husbands and children who don't currently participate in chores or shopping will thank you for this in the long run. What if something happened to you? What would hubby do if he had to handle these tasks himself? How would your children cope? Now, don't you feel better about delegating?

By delegating, you'll experience less stress in your life and you'll become more connected with your family and partner. You'll now have the time and the energy to exercise and your mood will be uplifted. Exercise is essential to good health – it's not a guilty pleasure and it's no doubt the best way to relieve stress and reduce weight. You'll become more energized and toned. You'll look and feel better and your confidence will sore. Studies reveal that when you feel more confident, you achieve more in life.

Now you can see why it's in *everyone's* best interest to stop and do something for YOU. Ask for help, and make time to go to the gym or take a walk, get a massage or pedicure, give yourself a mini-facial, read a book, or just relax and do nothing. Sharing responsibilities and taking "time-outs" for yourself will benefit your entire family.

Remember to acknowledge the help you get from your family while you enjoy your new found energy. Show appreciation and you'll soon find that they really don't mind helping. They may even volunteer!

You're Responsible for Your Own Happiness

Life is affected by the choices you make. You can make your life easy or difficult — it's entirely up to you. You are responsible for your own happiness and health. If you're unhappy with your weight, complexion, career, or relationship, it's your responsibility to address these issues. And YOU CAN do it!!! Begin by accomplishing one small thing each day to start your goal in motion. Visualize yourself achieving your goal and it will happen!

- If it's your goal to shed pounds, set aside a little time each day to exercise. Start by taking a walk with a co-worker or find a partner to join you at an exercise class. If you have someone counting on you, you'll likely stick with your exercise routine.

Exercise will help you feel uplifted, you'll become toned, diminish stress, and likely lose those stubborn pounds.
- Plan your diet by keeping healthy snacks handy. Snack on raw almonds or apple slices, herbal teas or lite cheese when you're at work. Take your lunch to work with you. You'll save money and you'll also control the portions and quality of food you eat.
- If you want a new job, prepare professional job resumes and mail one or two resumes each day. Make at least one to two daily phone calls that are directed toward finding your new job. Contact friends, relatives or acquaintances who may have contacts for you. Remember the expression, "If you don't ask for the order, you won't get it." By simply asking someone if they need help, you may find yourself in a terrific new job situation. You can make it happen.
- If it's your goal to improve your complexion, there are many easy, quick and affordable recipes, products and no-nonsense solutions listed throughout this book.

Just do *something* each day to keep your goal in motion. In no time, you'll begin seeing results and you'll find yourself looking forward to the next day and the next step toward your goal.

You will find practical, affordable, effective tips and suggestions throughout this book. Just flip through the Table of Contents to seek out your immediate concerns. You'll find skin and hair care tips, nail care suggestions, anti-aging, fitness and weight loss information, as well as product suggestions in the Best Beauty Buys lists following each remedy. There is something here for you, your partner, teenagers, friends, mother-in-law, sister....everyone. Of course, always check with your physician before starting a new diet, skin care regimen, or taking new supplements. Please read the "Disclaimer and Important Note to the Reader" before you begin.

Taking care of your personal needs will start you on a positive path to changing your life. You'll improve your career, likely lose those stubborn pounds, and maybe even add more romance to your life. Love yourself, embrace who you are, and take time for yourself because you're number one!!

Affordable Ways to Look 10 or More Years Younger

Yes, it's possible to non-invasively take years off your face and body! Wrinkles and aging **can** be prevented and even reversed. Keep your skin looking youthful, firm and nearly flawless with these highly effective, affordable methods:

1. Exfoliate (slough off) skin three or more nights a week. Frequent exfoliating stimulates collagen and elastin production, tightens and prevents sagging skin, diminishes pigmentation spots, reduces and repairs fine lines and can help thicken the skin. Women often avoid exfoliating the thinning skin of the temples, the neck, jowls and hands. These are the areas that can give away your age, so be sure to include them when exfoliating. Exfoliate three or more nights weekly and you'll begin to notice the skin on the temples thickening, the veins less protruding, the jowls becoming less droopy, the skin on the neck becoming tighter and age spots on hands and face fading. Exfoliating your body also helps keep skin more flawless-looking and firm. Exfoliate face, neck, jowls, temples, hands and body using either a), b), c) or d) exfoliating methods:

a) For normal, dry, mature, combination or oily skin:
After cleansing, while face is still wet, use a handful of baking soda to gently scrub face in a circular motion. Then rinse. Use

baking soda on a face cloth to exfoliate body (from neck to feet) in the shower. Baking soda is a mechanical exfoliant or scrub. Effective mechanical scrubs are now on the market. One of my favorites, a top seller, is Microdermabrasion Scrub. After just two to three uses, you'll see the same results as you would after having a costly microdermabrasion spa treatment. Apply to clean, wet face in a circular motion for about a minute. Then rinse. Over 30 treatments are in a jar. I also use baking soda or Microdermabrasion Scrub on my hands to keep them rejuvenated and smooth. See more products listed in the Best Beauty Buys below.

b) For oily, sun-damaged, sensitive or acne-prone skin exfoliate with a cream or liquid exfoliant: After cleansing, apply a cream that contains ingredients such as alpha lipoic, salicylic or glycolic acid or green tea extract. These ingredients can help brighten and gently exfoliate skin. Green tea has anti-bacterial properties that help keep blemishes in check. Alpha lipoic, salicylic or glycolic acid can help brighten and even skin tones. These are called cream exfoliants, which can also be used by those with rosacea.

c) *For sensitive, normal, dry or mature skin:*
After cleansing apply a Kinetin-based cream exfoliant. Kinetin acts like Retin-A to exfoliate skin but is more gentle. Aging Eraser by Age Advantage is a highly effective, gentle exfoliant and skin nourishing cream that's loaded with anti-oxidants and contains Kinetin. It's a popular choice of several soap and television stars. This is a cream exfoliant.

d) *Exfoliating Creams for all skin types*:
This past year, cutting-edge moisturizing and exfoliating creams have been developed. They are gentle alternatives to peels and

lasers. Products such as Relastyl™, Perfect RX Nite Serum and Perfect RX Beyond Essential Day Lotion contain Matrixyl, an active biopeptide that gently exfoliates, smoothes, helps brighten and thicken skin and helps diminish wrinkles by stimulating collagen over 300% and hyaluronic acid production over 200%. Matrixyl has been clinically proven to work more effectively than retinoids. Studies reveal after just three to six months, wrinkles and furrows are reduced by up to 68% and skin is more hydrated. Results are remarkable. Apply to face, neck, chest, under and around eyes and on hands. Apply daily with sunscreen overtop and nightly as a stand alone cream or with antioxidant-rich cream overtop. Matrixyl-based creams are safe to use on all skin types including skin of color. I also recommend that you use Microdermabrasion Scrub or baking soda nightly so creams will be even more effective.

2. Many antioxidant-rich creams contain effective, nourishing and anti-aging properties. They can help hydrate, protect against UV rays, help repair fine lines, fade pigmentation spots, tighten skin and calm inflammation. Apply them in the morning to face, neck, under eyes and on hands, followed by sunscreen overtop, then make-up. Or apply them at night. Read labels for antioxidant ingredients such as : Vitamin C or C-Ester, green or white tea extract, Astazanthin, Pycnogenol®, alpha lipoic acid, Vitamin A, Vitamin E or DMAE (derived from fish).

3. Antioxidant-rich Serums are more emollient than creams and are perfect for dry or mature skin. DMAE can help tighten and firm skin almost instantly.

4. Emu oil provides extra moisture for dry, mature or inflamed skin without clogging the pores. It is an anti-inflammatory too. Combine emu oil with moisturizer on the neck or under the eyes

where you'll likely need more moisture or need to diminish puffiness. Emu oil is reasonably priced and found in health food stores.

5. Hyaluronic acid creams and serums have recently become very popular because they can help tighten, plump and firm the appearance of skin. Hyaluronic acid can help improve collagen health for increased strength and elasticity, resulting in firmer-looking skin. Perfect for dry or mature skin.

6. Take years off your face, neck and hands and most likely avoid a face-lift with affordable, painless L.E.D. (Light Emitting Diode) Therapy. You'll be hearing more about L.E.D Therapy in the next few years as it will likely replace costly, painful laser resurfacing and face-lift surgery. L.E.D. Therapy is totally safe, painless, and can be used on ANY skin color or any age skin. L.E.D. emits wavelengths of light that help the body's ability to repair tissue. And it's affordable! Super Bright LED bulbs deliver warm heat and penetrate into the skin to stimulate the production of collagen, thus repairing and reducing the formation of wrinkles and can help prevent sagging skin. An increase of blood flow to the skin improves the skin tone and texture. Skin tightens and firms, pores become more refined, uneven skin diminishes. You'll notice broken capillaries diminishing, age spots fading, wrinkles disappearing and skin tightening in just six to eight treatments (sometimes even less). After just one treatment, rosacea flush can diminish. After six to eight treatments, simply do one treatment a month for maintenance. You can't over-use L.E.D. Therapy. It is also known to help increase blood flow to the scalp stimulating hair growth (if there is a viable follicle). It can also help diminish pain in the muscles, back, knees, hands, shoulders, and can relieve painful arthritis and aching joints. When you apply the unit to your hands to relieve painful arthritis,

you'll also rejuvenate them and help diminish age spots!! So many benefits. Both you and your spouse can use this remarkable, non-invasive therapy. Some California dermatologists and spas currently offer the treatment for about $65 to $125 a session. Great News — home units are now available! I've done my research and this one is a superior product. L.E.D. Therapy has been used by both NASA and the US Army to help quickly heal broken bones, sprains, wounds and more. Athletes have also been privy to it to quickly heal their injuries. Its anti-aging benefits have been clinically proven and documented.

Finally – a painless, safe, affordable and highly effective anti-aging alternative. Even better results are had when skin is exfoliated prior to treatment. Exfoliating face with Microdermabrasion Scrub or baking soda (see #1 above for instructions) will enhance the L.E.D. Therapy treatments as light can better penetrate. When combined with products containing Matrixyl or antioxidant-rich creams or serums, you'll most likely prevent a facelift. For more information on the home unit, email louisa@hollywoodbeautysecrets.com or call 1-877-568-4727.

7. Avoid sun exposure. Sun is responsible for 75% of wrinkles on your face, age spots on your hands, face and chest area. Did you know that skin damage can start after just ONE minute of exposure? Wearing effective sunscreen creates a barrier that causes sunlight to reflect away, preventing UV rays from penetrating into the skin. For full protection wear sunscreen every day - rain or shine. Sunscreen must be SPF 15 or higher. If you live in a sunny climate wear SPF 30. Read labels to ensure that your sunscreen contains ONE of the following effective ingredients to ensure full protection. Look for ingredients such as: Parsol®, avobenzene, zinc oxide or titanium dioxide. Choose sunscreen formulated for your skin type. Do

not use body sunscreen on your face. When outdoors wear a long sleeved shirt and sun visor for added protection. Wear cotton gloves to protect hands when driving as UV rays can penetrate through windshield glass. Mineral make-up also contains UV protection.

8. A daily antioxidant-rich supplement can help protect skin from free radical damage, and can help reverse the signs of aging and sun damage. Look for capsules that combine: Vitamin C or C-Ester, lipoic acid, DMAE (fish oil derivative), and Vitamin E. An additional 1000 mg. of Vitamin C, 60 mg Co-Q10, and drinking eight to 10 glasses of water daily are also recommended by anti-aging experts.

9. Daily flaxseed oil supplements can help slow down aging, hydrate skin, help ignite fat burning and can even help balance hormones. Lecithin can also help increase skin elasticity and thickness as well as improve hair and nail condition.

10. Yellow teeth and thinning lips can reveal your age. See the Lip and Oral Care section for quick and easy ways to brighten your pearly whites and naturally plump thinning lips.

11. Water can strip hands of moisture, cause splitting or peeling nails and is thought to be the cause of arthritis in joints of the hands. Wear lined rubber gloves when doing housework or dishes. Apply lotion frequently to hands.

12. Look and feel younger with anti-aging aglae, Sun Chlorella. This Japanese algae is the Hollywood beauty secret of many celebrities as well as many physicians. I also use it. Incredible anti-aging and nutrient-packed Sun Chlorella is a super toxin-fighter and immune-booster that is known to also help turn back

the clock and energize your body. Within weeks you'll have more energy and you'll see lines and wrinkles softening, age spots fading, pores tightening, smoother skin, improvement with dry skin or adult acne and you'll have a rosier, healthier complexion. It can also improve and strengthen nails and help hair become more shiny and soft. Sun Chlorella is a single-cell freshwater green algae that is a rich source of nucleic acid. It helps your body reproduce immune cells to help you feel energized and helps keep you youthful-looking.

Sun Chlorella can help alleviate digestion or stomach problems, can help prevent weight gain, can relieve joint pain and help fade pigmentation spots. Sun Chlorella can help your body renew itself by fighting off premature aging and contains 18 amino acids that protect your body's defenses. It includes cystine, T-cell building arginine and Lysine. Sun Chlorella can also:

- aid in clearing toxins, can assist weight loss and helps clear skin. When fat cells become clogged with toxins, the system becomes sluggish, constipated and weight gain is inevitable.
- help cleanse cells of fatigue-causing toxins that rob you of energy. You will have more energy and your mood will be uplifted.
- help increase oxygen to the cells. Many experience relief of asthma, fatigue, joint pain, stiffness and swelling.
- help keep your system regular because it contains the highest amount of chlorophyll.
- help prevent bad breath. Chlorophyll is the key.
- help protect your system from hormonal imbalances.
- help maintain healthy cholesterol levels, better circulation and blood pressure. For more information and **a free sample of Sun Chlorella, call 1-800-595-6776.** Let them know that Hollywood Beauty Secrets referred you.

13. Do not smoke. Smoking ages the face, body and hands, causes broken blood vessels, enlarged pores, pigmentation spots, lines around the mouth, crow's feet, a dull complexion and loss of elasticity in skin resulting in wrinkles. With this in mind, try to stop smoking. Try chewing gum or wear smokers' patches, which are formulated to help eliminate dependence on cigarettes. Hypnosis is another alternative that has helped many individuals. See resources for a top hypnotist who has helped hundreds of celebrities quit smoking including Matt Damon.

14. Many aspects of aging can be prevented or reversed when human growth hormone is naturally stimulated. By age 35 many of us exercise less and experience sleeplessness. When this happens, our natural production of growth hormone declines. When HGH production slows down we experience signs of aging such as gray hair, sagging skin, wrinkles, increased abdominal fat, cellulite, sleeplessness, loss of energy and libido, mood swings, depression, impaired vision, high cholesterol, thickening and hardening of the arteries and plaque formation. Weight resistance exercises and getting plenty of sleep can help increase the production of natural growth hormone in our bodies. Symbiotropin® is a popular natural blend of amino acids that is highly recommended by anti-aging therapists and doctors. It is not a steroid and is not human growth hormone. It's taken by millions.

15. Exercise is rejuvenating and probably THE best stress-reliever. And as we age, it's important to add weights or weight resistance exercise to our daily routine. This will ensure a more youthful, trim body. Weight resistance exercises stimulate the natural production of human growth hormone and help tone and tighten the body. When you exercise, you will also sleep better.

Try my personal "Under 30-Minute Model Sculpting Workout" available on DVD and VHS. These are the exercises that I have used throughout my 20 year modeling career. And all you need is a set of 3 lb. weights and a chair. In 30 minutes, you're done! Women have reported that it's one of the most challenging workouts ever and if you're short on time or can't get to the gym, these exercises target all problem areas for women.

16. Other popular exercise workouts in Los Angeles are Pilates, The Bar Method and Ashtanga Yoga. These effective, sculpting exercises define muscles, help flatten the abs, firm and lift buttocks, elongate legs, slim hips and tone arms. These workouts slightly differ, however all involve a series of controlled isometric or resistance movements that will have your body transformed within weeks. Because of its popularity, Pilates double, trio, and class rates are currently available. Now everyone can afford Pilates, not just celebrities. Beyond Physical Therapy in West Los Angeles offers several classes with superior instructors at discount rates for regulars and newcomers. I visited a few Pilates studios and what I enjoyed most about Beyond Physical Therapy is that it's a non-threatening environment, with serious instructors and you definitely see results – fast!! Even if you're a beginner, you'll feel at home there.

17. Limit use of alcohol. It dehydrates skin.

18. Minimize make-up. For youthful looking, glowing skin see my Anti-Aging 5-Minute Make-Up Application.

*BEST BEAUTY BUYS THAT CAN HELP YOU LOOK 10 OR
MORE YEARS YOUNGER*

L.E.D. Therapy Unit:
(To order contact louisa@hollywoodbeautysecrets.com)

Mechanical and Cream Exfoliants:
(To order visit www.hollywoodbeautysecrets.com)
- Microdermabrasion Scrub
- Aging Eraser by Age Advantage (with Kinetin)
- Perfect RX Nite Serum (with 8% Matrixyl)
- Perfect RX Beyond Essential Day Lotion (with 8% Matrixyl)
- Relastyl™ Deep and Fine Line Wrinkle Repair (Matrixyl)
- Perfect RX Beyond CP Lotion (for oily or acne-prone skin - contains salicylic acid)

(Available in your local grocery store)
- Baking Soda

Deep Wrinkle Diminishers:
(To order visit www.hollywoodbeautysecrets.com)

- Relastyl™ Deep and Fine Line Wrinkle Repair
- Perfect Rx Beyond Essential Day Lotion (8% Matrixyl)
- Perfect RX Nite Serum (8% Matrixyl)
(Available in your local drug store)
- Olay® Regenerist Serum

Serums:
(To order visit www.hollywoodbeautysecrets.com)

- Perfect RX Nite Serum (contains 8% Matrixyl)

Part One

- High Potency Vitamin C-Ester Serum (contains 45% C-Ester and Hyaluronic acid)
- DMAE Serum by Source Naturals

Antioxidant-Rich Creams:

(To order visit www.hollywoodbeautysecrets.com)
- Aging Eraser by Age Advantage
- DMAE-Alpha Lipoic-C-Ester Retexturizing Creme
- Alpha Lipoderm with Green Tea by derma e
- Astazanthin & Pycnogenol® Age Defying Nite Crème
- Hyaluronic Acid Day and Night Crème by derma e
- Hyaluronic Acid Firming Serum by derma e

Sunscreens:
(Available at your local drug store)

- Neutrogena ® UVA/UVB Sunblock, SPF 30 (Parsol)
- Banana Boat™ VitaSkin Advanced Sun Protection
- Oil of Olay Complete® (Zinc Oxide)

Other Products Recommended:
(To order visit www.hollywoodbeautysecrets.com)

- Symbiotropin (Human growth hormone stimulator) Receive a free copy of "Reversing Aging Naturally: The Methuselah Factor" by Dr. James Jamieson, Dr. L.E. Dorman with Valerie Marriott with your first order.

Videos:
(To order visit www.hollywoodbeautysecrets.com)

- Under 30-Minute Model Sculpting Workout (DVD & VHS)
- The Bar Method (double set)

Resources:

- L.E.D. Light Therapy:
Order home unit email louisa@hollywoodbeautysecrts.com
- Redlands, CA. Aesthetic Skin Care, 909-798-6766
- Connecticut, Anna Lamorte, 203-778-2858
- Honolulu, Wellness Institute, 808-941-6300
- Washington, Studio Donna Spa, 425-258-4941
- Colorado, Catherine's Skin Care, 303-377-6464
- New Jersey, Katherine's Aesthetics, 201-802-9300
- Encino, Epic The Salon, 818-716-8851
- Fountain Valley, Dr. E. Llorente, 714-885-8980

Pilates:

- Beyond Physical Therapy, Marina del Rey, CA. 310-578-5960. Receive 10% off when you mention Hollywood Beauty Secrets.

Hypnosis:

- Los Angeles, CA. Contact Kerry Gayner, 310-452-4256

Facial Care

• BATTLING BLEMISHES

To prevent blemishes, exfoliate your face regularly. Cleansers and moisturizers containing soy, salicylic, glycolic acid, sulfur or benzoyl peroxide can help prevent a breakout and unplug pores.

Apply ONE of the following remedies to blemishes at night. DO NOT COMBINE remedies as this may cause irritation.

1. Apply witch hazel to blemishes using a cotton swab. With the flip side of the swab apply calamine lotion. Let dry.

2. Apply milk of magnesia to blemishes using a cotton swab. Let dry. Magnesium is an anti-bacterial that absorbs oil.

3. Apply benzoyl peroxide to blemishes using a cotton swab. Let dry. With the flip side of the swab apply aloe vera gel.

4. Rub a clove of garlic or raw potato onto blemishes.

5. Apply egg yolk to blemishes using a cotton swab. Egg yolks are nature's natural Retin-A.

6. Apply saline eye drops to blemishes using a cotton swab. With the flip side of the swab apply milk of magnesia. Let dry.

7. Crush half an aspirin. Add a few drops of tea tree oil to make a paste and apply to blemishes.

8. Make a paste with ½ tsp. dry yeast and a few drops of tea

tree oil. Apply paste to blemishes.

9. Apply raw honey to blemishes using a cotton swab. Raw honey is a quick healer and natural antibiotic.

10. Apply ice, then hydrocortisone cream to large blemishes.

11. For an open blemish, apply witch hazel with a cotton swab. Let dry. Follow with antibiotic ointment. Witch hazel disinfects; antibiotic ointment speeds healing and prevents scarring.

12. Exfoliate (slough off skin) regularly to prevent plugged pores and blemishes. Exfoliate using Microdermabrasion Scrub or baking soda (mechanical scrub). After cleansing, while face is still wet, use a handful of baking soda to gently scrub face. Then rinse. Do not use mechanical scrubs on rosacea. Use a liquid or cream exfoliant.

13. Consuming zinc and soy-rich foods can help prevent blemishes and acne. Zinc-rich foods include eggs, liver, seafood, turkey, pork, mushrooms and milk. Soy-rich foods include soy milk (have a soy latte), soy yogurt, soy nuts, soybeans, soy cheese and tofu. You can also apply zinc ointment to blemishes. Dandellion root (tea) has been known to help purify the blood, which can help clear or prevent blemishes.

14. For quick healing apply a concealing stick containing salicylic acid on blemishes daily.

15. For a large, red blemish consider a high frequency treatment. Aestheticians use high frequency electrical current to kill blemish bacteria after a facial. The treatment is painless and offered at most skin care salons on a walk-in basis. It takes only

two to three minutes to zap stubborn blemishes. Within two days, the blemish is gone. It's usually free or just a couple of bucks if you walk-in without an appointment.

BEST BEAUTY BUYS FOR BATTLING BLEMISHES

Cleansers:
(To order visit www.hollywoodbeautysecrets.com)
- Glycolic Cleanser with Marine Plant Extracts
- Papaya and Soy Milk Foaming Face Cleanser
- BP (Benzoyl Peroxide) Pumice Cleanser

Blemish Fighting Creams:
(To order visit www.hollywoodbeautysecrets.com)
- Perfect RX Beyond CP
- Alpa Lipoderm with Green Tea Extract
- Aging Eraser by Age Advantage

(Available at your local drug store)
- Aveeno Skin Brightening Daily Moisturizer with Soy & Vitamins

Other Products Recommended:
(Available at your local drug store)
- Witch hazel
- Calamine Lotion
- Milk of Magnesia

Salicylic Acid Concealing Sticks:
(Available at your local drug store)
- Clean & Clear ® Concealing Treatment stick with salicylic acid

- Neutrogena ® Skin Clearing Oil-Free Concealer Salon Service:
- High Frequency is available at most skin care salons

• CAMOUFLAGING BLEMISHES

1. To quickly cover AND diminish blemishes, apply a tinted concealer containing salicylic acid. Choose a shade that is lighter than your foundation to conceal redness.

BEST BEAUTY BUYS FOR CAMOUFLAGING BLEMISHES

Salicylic Acid Blemish Concealers:
(Available at your local drug store)
- Maybelline ® Shine-Free Blemish Control Concealer
- Clean & Clear ® Concealing Treatment stick

• REMOVING BLACKHEADS & PREVENTING CLOGGED PORES

Exfoliate (slough off skin) three nights a week. This allows for easy blackhead removal, prevents clogged pores and stimulates collagen and elastin production. Below are several remedies to choose from:

1. Make a paste using 1 tbsp. baking soda, mixed with a few drops of water. In a circular motion, gently scrub face.

2. After just two uses of Microdermabrasion Scrub you will achieve similar results as you would after having a costly spa treatment. It contains crushed pearl powder and crystals to help unplug and exfoliate skin. Use it on hands too!

3. Add 1 tsp. Morton Salts and ½ tsp. hydrogen peroxide to ¼
cup boiled water. Let cool. Apply to face using a cotton pad.
Follow with the baking soda recipe above.

4. Bentonite clay is a deep pore cleanser that draws out
impurities and tightens skin. Mix equal parts of bentonite clay
and apple cider vinegar. Apply to blackheads. Let dry. Then
rinse with tepid water.

5. Natural fruit juices are excellent exfoliants. Apply tomato,
pineapple, lemon or grapefruit juice to blackheads using
a cotton pad. Wait five minutes. Rinse with tepid water.

6. Use a facial cleanser containing soy, glycolic or papaya
to help unplug pores.

*BEST BEAUTY BUYS FOR BLACKHEADS & CLOGGED
PORES*

Clog Eliminators:
(Available at your local health food store)
• Morton Salts
• Bentonite Clay
• Baking Soda

(To order visit www.hollywoodbeautysecrets.com)
• Microdermabrasion Scrub by derma e

Cleansers:
(To order visit www.hollywoodbeautysecrets.com)

- Glycolic Cleanser with Marine Plant Extracts
- Papaya and Soy Milk Foaming Face Cleanser
- BP (Benzoyl Peroxide) Pumice Cleanser

• TIPS TO HELP PREVENT ACNE

Acne and blemish breakouts can be due to low levels of zinc, Vitamin A or beta-carotene. High insulin levels in blood can also cause acne.

1. Consuming zinc-rich foods and taking zinc supplements (no more than 50 milligrams) daily can help keep acne in check. Zinc-rich foods include eggs, milk, liver, turkey, pork, soybeans, mushrooms, fish and shellfish. Vitamin A-rich foods include egg yolks and non-fat milk. Beta-carotene-rich foods include broccoli, tomatoes, watermelon, papaya, sweet potatoes, carrots, spinach and leafy, green vegetables. Soy-rich foods also prevent breakouts. They include tofu, soybeans, soy cheese, soy nuts, soy yogurt, shakes and soy milk. Dandelion root tea has been known to help purify the blood, which can help prevent blemishes.

2. High insulin levels in blood increase testosterone production, and stimulate the production of oil in the pores. The increased overgrowth of oil within pores causes clogging, infection and results in acne. Keep your insulin level low by eating a low-glycemic diet. Include protein, vegetables and fruits such as raspberries, strawberries, blackberries and blueberries. Avoid grains and starches such as bread, flour, pasta, potatoes, rice, corn, sugar, sweets, peas, beets, and high-glycemic fruits.

3. Medicated facial scrubs irritate acne and blemishes. Wash with liquid 2% salicylic acid (BHA) cleanser or ones that contain glycolic acid, soy, papaya or benzoyl peroxide. These types of cleansers unclog pores and gently exfoliate without irritating.

4. To prevent a breakout never touch your face with unwashed hands. Pull hair back when playing sports. Clean off cellular and home phones regularly using rubbing alcohol or a disinfecting wipe.

5. Moisturizers containing soy can balance oil gland production and prevent acne flare-ups.

6. A wonderful product called Skin and Pore Tightener is a 'mini-facelift' in a bottle! It includes 24K gold flakes, to strengthen skin's elasticity and firmness. The 24K gold flakes increase circulation in the skin which helps push out pollutants in the pores from the inside out. Skin/Pore Tightener revitalizes and tightens skin, minimizes lines around the mouth, frown lines on the forehead, and helps reduce the appearance of enlarged pores. Added green tea extract provides anti-inflammatory and anti-bacterial elements which help keep blemishes in check. Use on clean face before creams or make-up.

7. Moisturizers containing alpha lipoic acid and green tea extract reduce inflammation and enlarged pores. Green tea extract contains anti-inflammatory and anti-bacterial agents that help keep blemishes and acne in check.

8. Acne and Scar Crème contains regenerative properties that restore acne scars as well as burns, wounds or surgical scars. This revolutionary creme penetrates deep into the dermal skin

layer addressing scar tissue damage from the inside out and stimulates new cell growth. Glycolic acid is added to exfoliate and smooth the top layer of skin. Significant repair can be seen in 8 to 16 weeks.

9. Perfect RX Beyond CP is a new product that helps prevent acne, brightens skin and can help refine pores. It contains salicylic acid.

10. To camouflage large, red blemishes apply salicylic acid concealer stick daily. You may also consider a high frequency treatment to help quickly reduce a large blemish. Visit a local spa or see your aesthetician. High frequency takes just a minute or two and can be done on a walk-in basis. A treatment usually costs $5.00 or less.

11. Choose sunscreen, moisturizer and foundation formulated for oily or acne-prone skin.

12. Read more about laser and Blue Light Therapy for diminishing acne in "Anti-Aging Alternatives."

BEST BEAUTY BUYS TO PREVENT
ACNE AND BREAKOUTS

Cleansers:
(To order visit www.hollywoodbeautysecrets.com)
• Glycolic Cleanser with Marine Plant Extracts
• Papaya and Soy Milk Foaming Face Cleanser
• BP Pumice Cleanser (doctor formulated)

(Available at your local drug store)
• Neutrogena® Oil-Free Acne Wash

Blemish and Acne Creams:
(To order visit www.hollywoodbeautysecrets.com)
- Alpha Lipoderm & Green Tea Extract by Derma
- Acne and Scar Crème
- Perfect RX Beyond CP
- Skin & Pore Tightener by Age Advantage

Blemish Concealers:
(Available at your local drug store*)***
- Clean & Clear ® Concealing Treatment stick

● **RELIEVING ADULT ACNE**
Lower progesterone production may be the cause of
adult acne in women over age 30. See your physician or
dermatologist.

1. If you are NOT taking hormone replacement therapy,
applying topical natural progesterone cream or serum on acne-
prone areas may help. Natural progesterone cream can help
clear acne.

2. Lack of zinc may also cause acne. Consider zinc supplements
or zinc-rich foods such as eggs, liver, seafood, turkey, pork,
mushrooms, milk and soybeans. Vitamin A rich foods can help
reduce sebum or oils. You'll find Vitamin A in fruits, vegetables,
eggs and milk. Dandelion root tea has been known to help
purify the blood, which can help prevent breakouts.

3. Acne and Scar Crème contains regenerative properties
that restore acne scars as well as burn, wound or surgical scars.
This revolutionary creme penetrates deep into the dermal skin

layer addressing scar tissue damage from the inside out and stimulates new cell growth. Glycolic acid is added to exfoliate top layer of skin. Significant repair can be seen in 8 to 12 weeks.

4. Soy moisturizers can help prevent breakouts, brighten skin and can help fade pigmentation spots left by acne scars. You may also apply soy or plain yogurt with a squirt of lemon juice on your face. Let dry. Rinse with tepid water. Consume soy-rich foods such as tofu, soybeans, soy cheese, soy nuts, soy yogurt, shakes and soy milk.

5. Flax seeds contain phytoestrogens that can help balance hormones. Take flax seed oil supplements (capsules) or add ground flaxseeds to soups, protein shakes, tuna salad or dressing.

6. Sun Chlorella can help improve adult acne, helps diminish lines, wrinkles, age spots, helps smooth skin and tightens pores. It also helps detoxify the body and is recommended for its skin rejuvenating properties.

7. Choose foundation, sunscreen and moisturizer formulated for oily skin. During the day, instead of powdering oily areas, which traps debris on the skin, use rice blotting papers, a piece of a toilet seat cover or tissue curler papers to blot oil.

8. A wonderful product called Skin and Pore Tightener is a 'mini-facelift' in a bottle! It includes 24K gold flakes, to strengthen skin's elasticity and firmness. The 24K gold flakes increase circulation in the skin which helps push out pollutants in the pores from the inside out. Skin/Pore Tightener revitalizes and tightens skin, minimizes lines around the mouth, frown lines on

the forehead, and helps reduce the appearance of enlarged pores. Added green tea extract provides anti-inflammatory and anti-bacterial elements which help keep blemishes in check. Use on clean face before creams or make-up.

9. Blue Light Therapy can help dramatically reduce acne. Read more on Blue Light Therapy in "Anti-Aging Alternatives."

BEST BEAUTY BUYS FOR RELIEVING ADULT ACNE

(Available at your local health food store)
• Progesterone Serum and Creams

Foundations:
(Available at your local drug store)

• L'Oreal® Ideal Balance Foundation
• Maybelline® Shine-Free Oil Control Make-up

Oil-Blotting Papers:
(Available at your local drug store)
• Burt's Bees Wings of Love
• Clean & Clear® Oil Absorbing Sheets
• Toilet Seat Covers
• Hair Curler Tissues

Acne Products:
(To order visit www.hollywoodbeautysecrets.com)
• Skin & Pore Tightener by Age Advantage
• Acne and Scar Crème by Age Advantage
• Perfect RX Beyond CP Lotion

Other Products Recommended:
- Flax seeds and flax oil capsules, prices vary
- Sun Chlorella — for a free sample call 1-800-595-6776
- For more information on Blue Light Therapy, contact louisa@hollywoodbeautysecrets.com

- **PREVENTING A SHINY FACE**

Powder settles into fine lines on the face and can make skin look aged. For more youthful, shine-free skin absorb oil with one of the following:

1. Rice blotter papers.

2. A piece of toilet seat cover provides a quick oil blotting replacement.

3. Hair curler tissues are discreet and affordable oil blotters.

BEST BEAUTY BUYS FOR PREVENTING A SHINY FACE

Blotting Papers:
(Available at your local drug store)

- Lupia/Niplo Powder Papers (contain UV protection)
- Clean & Clear ® Oil Absorbing Sheets
- Toilet Seat Covers or Hair Curler Tissues

- **FACIAL MASKS**

For normal, dry, oily or mature skin, choose one of the following quick, effective mask recipes that best matches your skin type. If you feel any irritation, rinse the mask off immediately and follow with several splashes of cool water. Do not store these masks. Make each mask fresh.

- **FACIAL MASKS FOR OILY SKIN**

1. Mix 2 tbsp. lemon juice with 1 tbsp. bentonite clay. Apply to clean face for 20 minutes. Rinse with tepid water followed by a cool rinse. This mask draws out impurities and exfoliates.

2. Mix 2 tbsp. bentonite clay with 6 drops jojoba oil and two drops peppermint essential oil. Gradually add water to create a paste. Apply to clean face. Let set for 20 minutes. Rinse with tepid water followed by a cool rinse. This mask draws out impurities and stimulates circulation.

3. Combine 2 tbsp. plain yogurt with 1 tbsp. lemon or orange juice. Apply to clean face. Let dry. Rinse with tepid water followed by a cool rinse. This mask exfoliates, tightens and brightens skin.

4. Rub the inside peel of a papaya on face, neck, under eyes, and on hands. Let dry. Rinse with tepid water. Enzymes in papaya exfoliate, repair sun damage, diminish age spots and smooth skin. This mask is a natural alternative to Retin-A.

5. Apply 2 tbsp. soy yogurt on face. Soy brightens skin, fades pigmentation marks and exfoliates.

• FACIAL MASKS FOR DRY OR MATURE SKIN

1. Apply mayonnaise to clean face. Leave on for 10 to 15 minutes. Rinse with tepid water followed by a cool rinse. Vinegar and oil in mayonnaise exfoliate, brighten and moisturize skin.

2. Apply 2 tbsp. soy yogurt to clean face. Soy brightens skin, fades pigmentation marks and exfoliates.

3. Apply 1 tbsp. buttermilk to clean face for 15 minutes. Rinse with tepid water, followed by a cool rinse. This mask exfoliates, moisturizes and brightens skin.

4. Grind 1 tbsp. oatmeal in a blender and set aside. Add 1 tbsp. fennel seeds to ½ cup boiling water. Allow seeds to steep for 10 minutes. Strain seeds. Let liquid cool. Combine 1 tbsp. of liquid, ground oatmeal and 1 tbsp. honey. Apply to clean face for 20 minutes. Rinse with tepid water followed by a cool rinse. This mask moisturizes and heals skin.

5. Pour ½ cup boiling water over 3 tbsp. dried parsley. Allow to steep for 10 minutes. Strain the parsley. Let liquid cool. Mix 2 tbsp. ground oatmeal with 4 tbsp. of liquid. Mixture should have a paste consistency. Add more liquid or oatmeal if needed. Apply to clean face for 20 minutes. Rinse with tepid water followed by a cool rinse. This mask is soothing.

6. Rub the inside peel of a papaya on face, neck, under eyes, and on hands. Let dry. Rinse with tepid water. Enzymes in papaya exfoliate, repair sun damage, diminish age spots and smooth skin. This mask is a natural alternative to Retin-A.

7. Combine 2 tbsp. honey with 1 tbsp. apple cider vinegar or lemon juice. Apply to clean face for 20 minutes. This mask heals, moisturizes, brightens and exfoliates skin.

- **FACIAL MASKS FOR NORMAL SKIN**

1. Combine 2 tbsp. honey with 1 tbsp. apple cider vinegar or lemon juice. Apply to clean face for 20 minutes. Rinse with tepid water followed by a cool (not cold) rinse. This mask heals, exfoliates, brightens and moisturizes skin.

2. Apply 1 or 2 tbsp. fresh mashed avocado to clean face. Rub in a circular motion. Leave on face for 10 minutes. Rinse with tepid water followed by a cool rinse. This mask moisturizes skin.

3. Combine 2 tbsp. plain yogurt with 1 tbsp. lemon or orange juice. Apply to clean face. Let dry. Rinse with tepid water followed by a cool rinse. This mask brightens and exfoliates skin.

4. Apply mayonnaise to clean face. Vinegar and oil in mayonnaise exfoliates, brightens and moisturizes skin.

5. Rub the inside peel of a papaya on face, neck, under eyes, and on hands. Let dry. Rinse with tepid water. Enzymes in papaya exfoliate, repair sun damage, diminish age spots and smooth skin. This mask is a natural alternative to Retin-A.

- **FACIAL MASK FOR SUN BURNED SKIN**
Aloe gel is a known sun burn reliever. Both black and green tea contain tannic acid which is a natural anti-inflammatory agent. Place a black or green tea bag in a cup. Pour water over the bag. Let steep and then cool. Remove the tea bag and add 2 to 3 tbsp. of aloe vera gel. Stir, then apply mixture with a cotton pad or ball to sun burned areas. Leave on for 20 minutes or longer if you have time.

- **FACIAL MASK TO HELP FADE PIGMENTATION SPOTS**
Use this mask weekly to help fade pigmentation spots. Combine 3 tbsp. brown sugar, 1 tbsp. raw honey and 1 tbsp. fresh lemon juice in a small bowl. Cleanse face and gently scrub the pigmented areas first, then scrub entire face. Leave the mixture on your face for 3 to 5 minutes, then rinse with tepid water.

BEST BEAUTY BUYS FOR MASKS

- Ingredients listed are available at grocery and/or health food stores.

- **ANTI-AGING FACIAL EXERCISES**
Do these effective jowl and neck tightening exercises when you read or sit in front of the T.V. I do these when I'm in my car waiting at a stop light.

1. To do this jowl tightening exercise, pull your lips in and wrap them around your upper and lower teeth. The try to smile while lips are still in place and hold for 30 seconds, then repeat. This exercise tightens the jowls and muscles around the mouth.

2. To do this neck tightening exercise, curl your tongue back and hold while you roll your neck back. You may also pivot your head down and up from side to side. Great for tightening the neck and the jowls.

• FADING PIGMENTATION SPOTS & FRECKLES

Pigmentation spots, uneven skin tone and freckles are a result of sun exposure and/or hormone imbalances, contraceptives, childbirth or pregnancy. Exfoliating skin regularly can help keep pigmentation spots in check. Do not use Retinol (retinoids) or hydroquinone if pregnant, breast feeding or planning to become pregnant. Check with your doctor before using skin fading products or taking supplements. Here are some affordable and effective choices:

1. Exfoliate skin three nights a week. I recommend Microdermabrasion Scrub or exfoliating with baking soda. After cleansing apply either Microdermabrasion Scrub or baking soda on wet face using a gentle circular motion. Apply antioxidant-rich cream after exfoliating. Once a week, try the pigmentation facial mask in the previous mask section.

2. Look for skin care products that contain ingredients such as Pycnogenol®, Vitamin C, alpha hydroxy acid (AHA), Retinol (Vitamin A), soy, papaya, alpha lipoic acid, kojic acid, lactic acid, glycolic acid, orange or lemon juice and hydroquinone which can help fade pigmentation spots and brighten skin. See more details about these ingredients below:

• Pycnogenol®, a powerful antioxidant, was successfully tested and proven to significantly lighten over-pigmented areas like sunspots and melasma. Women who were given 75 mg. Pycnogenol® per day for one month, saw significant pigmentation reduction. Applying Pycnogenol® crème nightly or daily can protect the skin against free radicals and can help fade redness and/or pigmentation spots. **NOTE:** Check with your doctor before taking Pycnogenol® supplements. Pycnogenol creme can be safely used by those with rosacea.

- Topical Vitamin C is a powerful antioxidant that can help repair fine lines and wrinkles, helps protect skin from UV damage and can help fade pigmented spots. It contains anti-inflammatory agents.
- Alpha Hydroxy Acids exfoliate skin and can help fade pigmentation spots and even skin tones. AHA's also help unplug pores.
- Retinol (Vitamin A) is a prescription skin exfoliant that can help fade pigmentation spots and reduce lines and wrinkles. It can be irritating to those with sensitive skin.
- Kinetin can help gently brighten and even skin tone. It's as effective as retinol however, less irritating. Aging Eraser, a Kinetin-based antioxidant-rich moisturizer, is used by many television and soap stars. It helps brighten and even skin tones, exfoliates, nourishes and helps repair sun damaged skin.
- Kojic Acid and Hydroquonine are bleaching agents that help fade sunspots and melasma. These ingredients are combined in prescription skin fading creams.
- Soy and alpha lipoic acid can help gently fade pigmentation spots over time. You'll notice skin tones evening out in just two to three months.
- Lactic and glycolic acids are derived from milk or plants and found in many creams and cleansers. They can help brighten skin and fade pigmented areas.

- Plain or soy yogurt can help brighten and exfoliate skin. For more bleaching power, add 1 tbsp. fresh lemon or orange juice to either one. Apply to clean face. Let dry for 10 to 15 minutes. Then rinse with tepid water.

3. Sun causes pigmentation spots on the face. Rain or shine wear SPF 15 sunscreen specifically formulated for your skin type. Effective sunscreen must contain one of the following ingredients for full protection: Parsol®, avobenzene, titanium dioxide or zinc oxide.

4. For severe pigmentation spots wear additional sun screen over moisturizer. Apply SPF 30 sunscreen for added protection, especially if you live in a sunny climate. And wear a sun visor if spending any time outdoors.

5. One night a week, rub the inside of a papaya peel on face, under eyes and on neck. Enzymes in papaya exfoliate, repair sun damage, diminish pigmentation spots and help brighten and smooth skin. It's a natural alternative to Retin-A.

6. Try this mask weekly to help fade pigmentation spots. Combine 3 tbsp. brown sugar, 1 tbsp. raw honey and 1 tbsp. fresh lemon juice in a small bowl. Cleanse face and gently scrub the pigmented areas first, then scrub entire face. Leave the mixture on your face for 3 to 5 minutes, then rinse with tepid water. Lasts three days in the refrigerator.

7. This skin bleaching toner recipe works quite well. Combine the juice of ½ lemon and 3 oz. of witch hazel. Shake the mixture and apply bleaching toner to pigmented areas using a cotton ball or pad. Keep refrigerated for 5 days, then discard.

8. Wear a shirt with long sleeves and cotton gloves to protect skin from UV rays. Go walking after 5:00 p.m. or in the shade to prevent pigmentation damage.

9. Spot-Lite skin bleacher, developed by a dermatologist, can help fade pigmentation spots on face caused by exposure to the sun and hormones (freckles, age spots and melasma). Note: Spot-Lite contains hydroquinone.

10. A non-hydroquinone alternative that can help fade pigmentation spots is Skin Lighten & Age Spot Crème by Derma e. It contains licorice, milk thistle and Vitamin C for natural fading.

11. Acne and Scar cream contains glycolic acid which can help exfoliate scarred skin and stimulates new skin cell growth. It effectively fades pigmentation spots. Apply at night.

12. L.E.D. Therapy is an affordable, non-invasive and effective treatment that can help diminish pigmentation spots. No down time or pain is involved. Many celebrities are opting for L.E.D. Therapy as it is can help prevent wrinkles by stimulating collagen production. Purchase your own home L.E.D. Therapy unit. For more information about L.E.D. Therapy, see "Affordable Ways to Look 10 or More Years Younger" at the beginning of the book.

13. Intense Pulsed Light (IPL) Photofacials and can help fade freckles, port wine stains, rosacea and pigmentation spots, however it is very costly (approx. $250 - $550 a session) and generally five to six sessions are required to see results. IPL requires numbing cream. There is some down-time as treated

areas become darker for a several days so Light Therapy may be a better option.

14. Mineral make-up can nicely and naturally camoflauge pigmentation spots. I highly recommend Sheercover (TM) formulated by an aesthetician, Pauline Soli. See Beauty Buys.

BEST BEAUTY BUYS FOR FADING
PIGMENTATION SPOTS

Exfoliators:

(To order visit www.hollywoodbeautysecrets.com)
- Acne & Scar Crème by Age Advantage
- Micodermabrasion Scrub by Derma e
- Papaya Face & Soy Milk Mask By Derma e

Skin Lightening Antioxidant-Rich Creams:
(To order visit www.hollywoodbeautysecrets.com)
- Aging Eraser by Age Advantage
- DMAE, Vitamin C-Ester and Alpha Lipoic Acid Crème

Pigmentation Diminishers:
(To order visit www.hollywoodbeautysecrets.com)
- Spot-Lite™ by Age Advantage
- Pycnogenol® Moisturizing Crème with Vitamins C, E & A
- Skin Lighten & Age Spot Crème by derma e

(Available at your local health food store)
- Pycnogenol® Supplements

Facial Care

Sunscreen:
(Available at your local drug store)
- Neutrogena® UVA/UVB Sunblock (avobenzene)
- Oil of Olay® Complete (with zinc oxide) SPF 15
- Sheercover (TM) Mineral Makeup (UV protection). To order, call 1-800-506-6281.

Resources:
- L.E.D. Therapy:
Order home unit email louisa@hollywoodbeautysecrts.com
- Redlands, CA. Aesthetic Skin Care, 909-798-6766
- Connecticut, Anna Lamorte, 203-778-2858
- Honolulu, Wellness Institute, 808-941-6300
- Washington, Studio Donna Spa, 425-258-4941
- Colorado, Catherine's Skin Care, 303-377-6464
- New Jersey, Katherine's Aesthetics, 201-802-9300
- Encino, CA. Epic The Salon, 818-716-8851
- Fountain Valley, CA. Dr. E. Llorente, 714-885-8980

- **DIMINISHING NASAL HAIR**
Tweezing nasal hair can be uncomfortable and causes eyes and nose to water. Try either of these methods to rid nasal hair.
1. Applying baby teething ointment, or numbing cream containing lidocaine, on the inside of nostrils can help numb the area before tweezing. Wait 20 minutes. Then tweeze. If you don't have numbing cream, apply ice cubes to numb nostrils.
2. Clip nostril hair using cuticle scissors. You'll need a steady hand and a magnifying mirror.

BEST BEAUTY BUYS FOR DIMINISHING NASAL HAIR

(Available at your local drug store)
- Baby Teething Ointment
- Cuticle Scissors

• ANTI-AGING 5-MINUTE MAKE-UP APPLICATION
When you've got just five minutes to get ready, try this quick and effective anti-aging make-up application. You'll look fresh and dewy in no time.

1. If you're prone to eye puffiness in the morning, at night before bed apply a drop of emu oil under eyes. Emu oil can help diminish inflammation in about 7 to 10 days. Apply serum such as Perfect RX Beyond Nite Serum or High Potency Vitamin C Ester Serum to face, under eyes and on neck.

2. In the morning after cleansing, apply an illuminating facial moisturizer, Relastyl™, or Aging Eraser on face, under eyes, on crow's feet and neck.

3. Next apply sunscreen.

4. Spread a pea-sized amount of sheer or illuminating foundation on each cheek, the forehead, and chin. Blend well over entire face and down the neck. Avoid applying on crow's feet if you have them, as this can accentuate lines. Mineral make-up is an another alternative to liquid foundation. It blends beautifully, especially on dry or mature skin and helps minimize the look of wrinkles, covers blemishes, pigmentation spots, or melasma.

Minerals also contain natural UV protection. Great for all skin types. I love mineral make-up for everyday wear.

5. Apply illuminating concealer from inner corner of the eyes to the center under the eyes. Then apply illuminating concealer just under the brows to highlight eyes. And apply a dab of illuminating concealer on the center of the eye lids. This highlights the eye.

6. Apply stick or cream blush to apples of cheeks and blend well. Dab a little blush at the base of the brow bone and blend. If you prefer powder blush first apply translucent powder to cheeks and oily T-zone only. Then apply powder blush.

7. Lightly pencil in brows if needed. Valerie of Beverly Hills makes a great universal brown color for all brows.

8. For a fresh, natural open-eyed look, draw a line of baby pink soft pencil shadow under the eyebrow and blend it in. Your eyes instantly open with this simple beauty trick. I also apply the baby pink pencil in the dark areas by the nose. Valerie of Beverly Hills makes a superior baby pink pencil (Naturelle), which I use and highly recommend. She's sold thousands.

9. Curl lashes using an eyelash curler. Apply one coat of mascara to top lashes only. Apply a second coat only on the outer third lashes, for more lengthy looking lashes. I'm often asked what mascara I use. I highly recommend Maybelline® Sky High Curves. This is my absolute favorite mascara, without a doubt! It lengthens and curls my lashes and does not smudge. Easy to remove too.

10. Lip gloss looks more youthful than lipstick. Try a flesh or berry-tinted lip gloss. Avoid lip liner. Glossy, unlined lips appear fuller than lined lips.

11. DO NOT apply powder as it settles into fine lines (unless you're using mineral make-up which comes in a powder form). Instead, blot face throughout the day using rice blotting papers, hair curler tissue paper or a piece of toilet seat cover.

12. For makeup application lessons, contact Sandra Marshall at 818-225-1874 or 818-448-5144. For camoflauge makeup, contact Sue Sigrist at 310-301-0363.

BEST BEAUTY BUYS FOR ANTI-AGING 5-MINUTE MAKE-UP APPLICATION

Anti-Aging Creams:
(To order visit www.hollywoodbeautysecrets.com)
• Relastyl™ Deep and Fine Line Wrinkle Repair
• Perfect Rx Nite Serum
• Age Eraser by Age Advantage

(Available at your local health food store)
• Emu Oil

Moisturizers with Effective Sunscreen:

(Available at your local drug store)
• Aveeno® Skin Brightening Daily Moisturizer
• Olay Complete® UV Protective Moisture Lotion

Just Sunscreen:
(Available at your local drug store)
- VitaSkin® Advanced Sun Protection (with avobenzene)
- Neutrogena® UVA/UVB Sunblock (with avobenzene)

Foundation Make-up:
(Available at your local drug store)
- Revlon® Skinlights Diffusing Tint SPF 15
- L'Oreal® Translucide Naturally Luminous Make-Up
- Maybelline Smooth Result® Age Minimizing Make-Up
- Neutrogena® Healthy Skin Liquid Make-Up SPF 20 (normal to oily skin)
- Cover Girl ®Smoothers All Day Hydrating Make-up (normal to oily skin)

Mineral Make-Up:
- Sheercover (TM) Mineral Makeup. To order call 1-800-506-6281

Illuminating Concealers:
(Available at your local drug store)
- Cover Girl® Illuminator
- Clean & Clear® Under Eye Brightening Stick Blush
- Cover Girl® Cheekers Blush (Pretty Pink)
- Maybelline® Express Blush

Universal Brow Pencils:
(These excellent pencils can be used on all brow colors)
- Brow Queen Pencil by Valerie of Beverly Hills (Bunny). To order call 1-800-282-5372.
- Brenda Christian Brow Pencil

Pink Hi-Liter Pencil:
- Naturelle Hi-liter Pencil by Valerie of Beverly Hills (Naturelle). To order call 1-800-282-5372.

Mascara:
(Available at your local drug store)
- Maybelline® Sky High Curves
- L'Oreal® Waterproof Mascara
- L'Oreal® Voluminous Mascara

Lip Gloss:
(Available at your local drug store)

- Sally Hansen® Lip Moisturizer (Clear Buff, Mauve or Nude)
- Cover Girl® Lipslicks
- Burt's Bees® Lip Shimmer

Oil Absorbing Sheets:
(Available at your local drug store)
- Burt's Bees® Wings of Love
- Clean & Clear® Oil Absorbing Sheets
- Toilet Seat Covers

(Available at your beauty supply shop)
- Hair Roller Tissues

Special Skin Needs

- **RELIEVING ROSACEA**

Those who suffer from rosacea may greatly benefit from the following remedies listed below. However, consult with a dermatologist first.

1. Cleanse skin with liquid 2% salicylic acid cleanser. This gentle cleanser reduces inflammation and redness without irritating skin.

2. Applying topical Pycnogenal® cream or gel can benefit the capillary system and help reduce redness and inflammation associated with rosacea. Alpha lipoic acid and green tea extract moisturizer is also a beneficial cream.

3. Scrubbing, rubbing, using abrasive exfoliants or wash cloths exacerbates rosacea. Never use these exfoliants.

4. Vitamin B-12 injections have been know to help remedy rosacea.

5. Avoid saunas, sun exposure, cold winds, hot tubs, exfoliants, smoking, stress, spicy or hot foods, and hot beverages as these will likely trigger an outbreak.

6. Avoiding sour cream, yogurt, chocolate, soy sauce, vinegar, navy beans, lima beans, pea pods, spinach, eggplant, tomatoes, bananas, citrus fruits, raisins, plums, figs and liver can help prevent outbreaks.

7. Recommended foods include antioxidant-rich vegetables such as broccoli, artichokes, asparagus, green beans, leafy lettuces and fruits such as blueberries, raspberries, strawberries, blackberries, peaches, plums and cantaloupe.

8. Avoid alcohol (red wine, vodka, gin, beer, champagne and bourbon) hot coffee, hot cider, hot chocolate and tea.

9. Avoid cosmetics and products containing fragrance, alcohol, peppermint, witch hazel, menthol, Retinoids (Retin-A, Renova) and facial masks.

10. Zinc (50 mg.) and Vitamin A (10,000 I.U.) daily can help minimize rosacea.

11. Mineral makeup can help camoflauge redness associate with rosacea.

12. Just one session of Light Therapy can help diminish the red flush of rosacea. It's also anti-aging, helps diminish wrinkles, tightens skin, help refine pores and can help fade pigmentation spots. See more on Light Therapy in "Affordable Ways to Look 10 or More Years Younger" at the beginning of the book.

13. A series of IPL Photofacials can help diminish rosacea and pigmentation problems, however it can be costly at about $250 to $500 a session and usually five to six sessions are required.

BEST BEAUTY BUYS FOR ROSACEA

(Available at your local drug store)
- Neutrogena® Acne Wash (contains 2% salicylic acid
- Zinc and Vitamin A supplements

(To order visit www.hollywoodbeautysecrets.com)
- Glycolic Cleanser with Marine Plant Extracts
- Pycnogenal ® Crème or gel with Vitamin C, E & A by Derma e
- Alpha Lipoderm Alpha Lipoic with Green Tea Complex by Derma e

Other Recommendations:

- Visit www.rosacea.org for more information
- Sheercover(TM) Mineral Makeup, call 1-800-506-6281

(To order visit www.hollywoodbeautysecrets.com)
- Light Therapy Home unit

- **RELIEVING ECZEMA**
This skin disorder causes inflamed, red areas or dry patches on the skin. Wind, extreme temperatures, hot or cold water, anxiety and stress may trigger an outbreak of eczema. Consult a dermatologist.

1. Taking borage and flaxseed oil supplements three times daily can help ease eczema. Essential fatty acids (EFA) supplements combine borage, flax and fish oil.

2. Eliminate or reduce dairy. Soy, goat or sheep cheeses are preferable substitutes. Shellfish, sugar, yeast, strawberries and pineapple may exacerbate eczema.

3. Drinking teas containing honey, ginger or chamomile can calm eczema. Foods such as peas, snow peas, split pea soup

and ginger soup are good choices for calming eczema. This Chinese tonic is known to help: Add 2 tbsp. bee pollen, 2 tbsp. raw honey, 1 tbsp. ginseng extract to a cup of hot water. Stir and drink each morning. You can find bee pollen and ginseng extract at your local health food store.

4. Temporarily clear dry patches with Hydrocortisone cream.

5. Fatty acids in oatmeal moisturize dry skin and reduce inflammation. Oatmeal lotions and/or oatmeal baths offer immediate relief.

6. 2% salicylic acid cleanser gently exfoliates (sloughs off) dry skin without irritation. Witch hazel can also help calm eczema.

7. Stress may also trigger an outbreak. Try Rescue Remedy Oral Spray when you're stressing out.

8. Bee pollen and honey are known to help eczema. Try Egyptian Magic All-Purpose Healing Cream. This word-of-mouth phenomenon contains bee pollen, honey as well as other natural moisturizing agents that can relieve the itchy, dryness associated with eczema.

9. Dandelion root tea is a blood purifier that can help with psoriasis and eczema. Milkthistle can also help relieve eczema as well as detoxify the liver. It can also help balance hormones. Check with your doctor before taking supplements.

10. Nanak's All-Natural Skin Repair works wonders on dry eczema patches.

BEST BEAUTY BUYS FOR ECZEMA
(To order visit www.hollywoodbeautysecrets.com)
- Egyptian Magic All- Purpose Healing Cream

(Available at your local health food store)
- Total EFA by Health From the Sun
- Flaxseed oil capsules and Flax seeds
- Bee Pollen
- Honey
- Ginseng Extract
- Rescue Remedy Oral Spray
- Nanak's All-Natural Skin Repair

(Available at your local drug store)
- Hydrocortisone Cream
- Neutrogena® Acne Face Wash (with 2% salicylic acid)
- Aveeno® Daily Moisturizing Lotion

- **RELIEVING PSORIASIS**
This disorder causes inflammation, scaling, flaky, itchy patches on skin. Consult a dermatologist.

1. Applying natural, topical progesterone cream on red, scaly patches can help relieve psoriasis. Progesterone cream is risk-free and eliminates most symptoms. Many cases of remission have been reported with its use. Do not use progesterone cream if taking hormone replacement therapy (HRT's). Check with your doctor before using progesterone cream.

2. Daily application of Vitamin C-Ester reduces redness and

scaling associated with psoriasis. Applied daily, many improvements are see within three to four months use.

3. Archives of Dermatology reports that fungus living in the lesions on the skin may cause psoriasis. Sugar stimulates production of fungus. Avoid sugar, high-glycemic foods such as candy, soft drinks, ice cream, cereal, pastries, pudding, pasta, bread, rice, pasta, rolls, green peas, corn, beets, bananas, potatoes and grains. Choose low-glycemic fruits such as blueberries, cantaloupe, raspberries, strawberries, kiwi, papaya and watermelon. Choose vegetables such as dark and leafy greens, celery, red and green peppers, Brussel sprouts, broccoli, cabbage, radishes, tomatoes and turnips.

4. Oil of oregano's anti-fungal and antibacterial properties relieve lesions, inflammation, itching, swelling and soreness. Apply oil on lesions twice daily. Pour three to four drops of oil of oregano into a gelatin capsule and take one capsule daily with meals.

5. Wash with 2% salicylic acid cleanser to reduce flaky, dry patches.

6. Taking a flax-primrose combination with borage oil can help relieve psoriasis.

7. Milk Thistle can help relieve psoriasis as well as detoxify the liver and balance hormones. Check with your doctor before taking supplements.

8. Egyptian Magic All-Purpose Healing Cream is known to help relieve the dry patches associated with psoriasis.

BEST BEAUTY BUYS FOR PSORIASIS

Products Recommended:
(**To order visit www.hollywoodbeautysecrets.com**)
- Egyptian Magic All- Purpose Healing Cream
- High Potency Vitamin C-Ester Serum

(Available at your local health food store)
- Flax Seeds, Flax-Primrose Combo and Borage oil
- Oil of Oregano. To order call 800-243-5342.

(Available at your local drug store)
- Neutrogena Acne Wash (2% salicylic acid)

- **RELIEVING KERATOSIS PILARIS** ("Chicken Skin Bumps")

Perhaps you or someone you know is challenged with rough, sometimes sandpaper-like red bumps that are most frequently scattered along the upper arms and thighs. Cheeks, back and buttocks can also become affected at one time or another. These bumps can be annoying, unsightly, chronic, sometimes even embarrassing and very common. Keratosis Pilaris is hereditary and affects 50% of the world's population. While this condition seems more pronounced at puberty, it frequently improves with age and tends to be less active during the summer. Keratosis pilaris may not be curable because it is genetically predetermined. However, treatments do exist to improve the skin affected. Excess skin cells build up around individual hair follicles. The normal shedding of old skin cells does not occur effectively as new cells are formed, giving the appearance of raised, rough, bumpy and uneven texture. Embarrassing pinpoint red or brown spots can develop beneath inflamed hair follicles because keratin scales prevent hair from reaching the surface. Regular exfoliating can help. Washing with cleansers containing glycolic or salicylic acid can help. Lotions containing and lactic acid, Vitamin C, Urea and Retin-A can be applied afterward. Regular microdermabrasion can also provide results. Microdermabrasion Scrub or simply some baking soda on a wet face cloth or loofa can be rubbed on the bumpy areas. You may also consider a light chemical peel. See your dermatologist.

BEST BEAUTY BUYS FOR KERATOSIS PILARIS

(To order visit www.hollywoodbeautysecrets.com)
• Glycolic Facial Wash with Marine Plant Extracts
• PB Pumice Scrub
• Microdermabrasion Scrub by derma e

Resources:
Chemical Peel
• Fountain Valley, CA. Dr. E. Llorente, 714-885-8980
• Redlands, CA., Aesthetic Skin Care, 909-798-6766

Eye Care

- **EFFECTIVE EYE CREAMS**

Below are some of the most effective eye creams I've come across. These products can help smooth, tighten and diminish fine lines and wrinkles as well as help fade dark circles and puffiness. If you are hesitant to try costly, painful wrinkle-reducing injections, consider one of the following:

1. A wonderful cutting-edge eye product called Perfect RX Eye Serum is to date the only product I've found that contains 8% Matrixyl which helps stimulate collagen over 300% and hyaluronic acid production over 200%. Matrixyl is clinically proven to be more effective than Retinol and can help dramatically diminish fine lines and wrinkles. Perfect RX Eye Serum also contains Vitamin K and Haloxyl to help effectively fade dark circles, DMAE to firm the eye area, and Alpha Lipoic Acid to help diminish puffiness and brighten the eye area. A superior all-in-one product for the eyes. It's developed by a board certified anti-aging expert and registered nurse. It's best worn daily. At night wear Ultimate Eye Cream or an antioxidant-rich cream like Pycnogenol® Age Defying Nite Crème.

2. Relastyl™ Deep and Fine Line Wrinkle Repair also contains Matrixyl (4%) and can be worn under and around eyes and on the entire face and neck.

3. Ultimate Eye Crème™ by Age Advantage can help diminish puffiness, dark circles and fine lines. It contains DMAE, alpha lipoic acid, Vitamin K, emu oil and other anti-oxidants which penetrate deep into the cells creating smoothness, firming,

elasticity and can help diminish dark circles. Emu oil assists the nourishing ingredients to penetrate into the skin and helps diminish puffy eyes. Ultimate Eye Crème is best worn at night, but many individuals are known to wear it in the day too.

4. Aging Eraser™ by Age Advantage, a Kinetin-based facial cream, also contains DMAE, Vitamin A, CoQ10 and emu oil. This face cream can be safely worn under the eyes. Kinetin acts like Retin-A to gently exfoliate skin and help diminish fine lines without dryness or irritation. DMAE firms the skin and can be worn on its own or over Vitamin-C Ester serum at night.

5. Antioxidant-rich serum, High Potency Vitamin C Ester Serum™ contains the highest amount of C-Ester (45%), combined with anti-aging hyaluronic acid, which keeps the eye area hydrated and repairs fine lines. Wear serum alone on clean skin or you can also top it with antioxidant-rich eye cream for extra moisture and nourishment at night.

6. To relieve puffiness under eyes as well as moisturize dry, mature skin around eyes, combine a drop or two of emu oil with any eye cream. You may also wear emu oil on its own.

7. StriVectin-SD™ a stretch mark cream, has been known to help diminish fine lines around the eyes.

8. Light Therapy is also highly recommended to help reduce fine lines and wrinkles around the eyes.

BEST BEAUTY BUYS FOR EYE CREAM

Creams for Eyes:
(To order visit www.hollywoodbeautysecrets.com)
- Perfect RX Eye Serum
- Relastyl™ Deep and Fine Line Wrinkle Repair
- Ultimate Eye Crème™ by Age Advantage
- Aging Eraser™ by Age Advantage
- StriVectin-SD™

Serums:
(To order visit www.hollywoodbeautysecrets.com)
- High Potency Vitamin C Ester Serum (45% Vitamin C-Ester)
- Perfect RX Eye Serum

Other Products Recommended:
(Available at your local health food store)
- Emu Oil

- **DIMINISHING DARK CIRCLES**
1. A wonderful product called Perfect RX Eye Serum contains Matrixyl to stimulate collagen and hyaluronic acid, Vitamin K and Haloxyl to dramatically fade dark circles, DMAE to firm the eye area as well as Alpha Lipoic Acid to help diminish puffiness and brighten the eye area. A superior all-in-one product for the eyes, created by a board certified anti-aging expert and RN.

2. Ultimate Eye Cream is another popular choice as it contains DMAE, alpha lipoic acid, emu oil to help diminish puffy eyes,

Vitamin K to help fade dark circles and antioxidants to help nourish and help repair fine lines.

3. Apply potato slices on closed eyes for 5 minutes. Enzymes help fade redness and puffiness.

4. Apply an effective crease-free concealer to camouflage dark circles.

5. Light diffusers in illuminating concealers brighten and open tired looking eyes. Apply illuminating concealer on the inside corners of eyes and in the dark areas next to the nose to create brighter eyes. One of my favorites and that of dozens of models and make-up artists, is Touche Eclat by Yves St. Laurent. This is the only department store product I recommend because it's simply amazing. It's a highlighter and dark circle corrector that costs about $35 but lasts forever! Mine lasted about 11 months. Truly worth every penny as it does not crease and beautifully covers darkened areas in the corners and under the eyes.

6. Also recommended are Valerie of Beverly Hills Naturelle Hi-Liter Pencil and Cover Girl® Illuminating Stick.

BEST BEAUTY BUYS FOR DARK CIRCLES

Effective Eye Creams:

(To order visit www.hollywoodbeautysecrets.com)
• Perfect RX EyeSerum
• Ultimate Eye Creme by Age Advantage

(Available in your local health food store)
• Vitamin K 7 Oils & 7 Herbs Crème, Orjene® Organics

- Vitamin K Cream By Reviva® Labs

Crease-Free Concealers:

(Available at your local drug store)
- L'Oreal® Visible Lift Line Minimizing Concealer
- Almay® Skin-Smoothing Concealer with Kinetin
- Yves St. Laurent™ Touche Eclat Radiant Touch (Available at department stores)
- Valerie of Beverly Hills Naturelle Hi-Liter. To order call 1-800-282-5374.

Illuminating Concealer:
- Cover Girl® Illuminator Concealer Stick
- Valerie of Beverly Hills Naturelle Hi-Liter Pencil. To order call 1-800-282-5374

• DIMINISHING PUFFY EYES
1. Emu oil is an emollient containing anti-inflammatory agents that reduce puffiness. Apply under eyes nightly or sparingly during the day. Emu oil can be worn over any eye cream. It does not clog pores. Ultimate Eye Crème effectively minimizes puffiness, and dark circles. It contains emu oil and many anti-oxidant ingredients. You'll notice puffiness diminishing in seven to 12 days.

2. A wonderful product called Perfect RX Eye Serum is probably the only product I've found that contains Matrixyl to stimulate collagen and hyaluronic acid as well as Alpha Lipoic Acid to help diminish puffiness, Vitamin K and Haloxyl to dramatically fade dark circles, and DMAE to firm the eye area and help diminish puffy eyes.

3. Alpha lipoic acid and green tea extract cream can help reduce puffy eyes and dark circles.

4. Chamomile, green and black tea contain tannins that have anti-inflammatory properties. Apply two cool, wet tea bags on closed eyes for 10 to 15 minutes.

5. Apply egg whites under eyes. Let dry. Egg whites can help tighten loose skin.

6. Place cucumber slices on closed eyes for five minutes.

7. Gently rub the juice of a slice of raw potato under the eyes. The enzymes in the juice diminish puffiness in about 10 minutes. Rinse, dry, then apply eye cream.

8. Hemorrhoid cream is known to help decrease blood supply to the eye area which can help reduce puffiness.

9. Try sleeping with two pillows at night to help keep head elevated. This prevents fluid from settling around the eyes.

10. Cut back on liquids before bed as this may increase puffiness around the eyes in the morning. Drink more fluids during the day.

BEST BEAUTY BUYS FOR PUFFY EYES

(To order visit www.hollywoodbeautysecrets.com)
- Ultimate Eye Crème by Age Advantage
- Perfect RX Eye Serum

Eye Care

- Alpha Lipoderm Alpha Lipoic Acid with Green Tea extract

(Available at your local health food store)
- Emu Oil
- Green or Chamomile tea

• TWEEZING EYEBROWS
1. To relieve the discomfort of tweezing apply baby teething ointment or lidocaine numbing cream to brows 20 minutes before tweezing. If you don't have numbing cream, ice cubes can help numb brows.

2. For precision tweezing, try Tweezerman® tweezers. The precision angle can grab the finest, shortest hairs.

3. For sparse or bare patches throughout the brows consider taking silica gel and/or prenatal vitamins and applying topical WEL Scalp Stimulator. This combination is known to help brow hair grow in.

4. Valerie of Beverly Hills offers a variety of brow stencils and pencils or powders that are simply the best. To order, call 1-800-282-5374.

5. Permanent makeup can help fill in sparse brows. See more about permanent makeup in "Anti-Aging Alternatives".

BEST BEAUTY BUYS FOR TWEEZING BROWS

(Available at your local beauty supply store)
- Tweezerman® Tweezers

(Available at your local health food store)
- Silica Gel
- Prenatal Vitamins

(To order visit www.hollywoodbeautysecrets.com)
- WEL Scalp Stimulator

Lip & Oral Care

• ELIMINATING BAD BREATH

1. Drinking green tea can help banish bad breath. It's more effective than chewing gum or mints.

2. Floss teeth once or twice daily. Scrape your tongue with a teaspoon each morning to remove bacteria. Scrape from back of the tongue forward. Store flossing sticks in your purse or in a small zip-lock bag for convenience at work or when traveling.

3. Chewing on fennel seeds after eating a meal or snack can help eliminate bad breath. Swallow or discard seeds after chewing.

4. Dental whitening gum contains baking soda which can fight bad breath.

5. Gum disease can cause bad breath. See your dentist.

6. Myrrh is an effective oral antiseptic. Make a mouthwash combining 4 or 5 drops of myrrh essential oil in a cup of mint tea and use as mouthwash.

7. Sun Chlorella is loaded with chorophyll which can effectively help eliminate bad breath. It has many other anti-aging and health benefits as well. Read more about sun chlorella in "Affordable Ways to Look 10 or More Years Younger" at the beginning of the book.

Part Five

BEST BEAUTY BUYS FOR ELIMINATING BAD BREATH

(Available in your local drug store)
- Flossing sticks
- Whitening Gums

(Available in your local health food store)
- Myrrh Egyptian Oil
- Sun Chlorella
- Green Tea

• RELIEVING CHAPPED, CRACKED LIPS
Lips can easily become dehydrated due to exposure to sun, wind, cold and heat. As lips do not have oil glands they are vulnerable to dryness and becoming cracked, chapped or red. Below are some effective remedies that can help smooth lips:

1. Exfoliate (slough off) and moisturize lips to keep them nourished and line free. Twice a week dab milk-saturated cotton pads on lips for three minutes. Rinse then apply Vitamin E, castor oil or petroleum jelly. Milk contains lactic acid which exfoliates dry skin. The fat in milk moisturizes.

2. Apply raw, unpasteurized honey to lips and top with Vitamin E, petroleum jelly or castor oil. Leave on overnight. Raw honey helps smooth and heal peeling, chapped lips. Vitamin E heals and moisturizes. Petroleum jelly and castor oil seal in moisture.

3. To soften and smooth lips, combine 1/4 tsp. honey, ¼ tsp. lemon juice and ½ tsp. Vitamin E oil. Leave on lips overnight.

4. Apply a wet, warm, black tea bag on dry or cracked lips. Black tea contains tannins that soften, moisturize and heal chapped or cracked lips.

5. To smooth chapped lips, mix 1 tsp. baking soda with a few drops of water to make a paste. In a gentle, circular motion rub lips. Follow with Vitamin E, castor oil or petroleum jelly.

6. Choose lip balms and lip sticks that contain SPF 15 and hydrating ingredients such as cocoa and shea butter, honey, beeswax, glycerine, castor, primrose, olive or almond oil. Egyptian Magic is an all-purpose healing balm that contains honey as well as other healing ingredients. Egyptian Magic helps smooth and heal chapped, cracked lips, help calm rashes, blemishes, heal burns and more. Buzz Lip Honey is another honey and wax based stick that helps soothe chapped lips.

7. The wax base of Chapstick® provides an excellent base for smooth lipstick application. It also helps protect lips from chapping with its smooth coating.

8. Burt's Bees ® Lip Shimmer provides UV protection and is available in a nice assortment of colors that contain Vitamin E and titanium dioxide.

9. Nanak's All-Natural Skin Repair is a new find. It makes my lips rosy and moisturizes.

Part Five

BEST BEAUTY BUYS FOR RELIEVING CHAPPED LIPS

(To Order visit www.hollywoodbeautysecrets.com)
- Egyptian Magic All-Purpose Healer

(Available at your local health food store)
- Buzz Lip Honey Stick
- Burt's Bees® Lip Shimmer
- Chapstick®
- Blistex® Herbal Answer
- Nanak's All-Natural Skin Repair

• SMOOTHING LINES AROUND THE MOUTH
1. To diminish lines around the mouth, exfoliate regularly. Here are some affordable and effective methods:
a) Rub the inside peel of a ripe papaya around mouth and on lips. The moisture left on your skin will dry in about 10 to 15 minutes. Then rinse. Enzymes in papaya exfoliate, help repair sun damage and smooth skin. Papaya is a natural alternative to Retin-A. Top skin care salons charge $65 to $85 for papaya enzyme masks. Do this yourself for $2.
b) Apply baking soda to wet face in a gentle, circular motion, focusing on the fine lines around the mouth. Then rinse.
c) Microdermabrasion Scrub is another popular choice. It contains crushed pearl powder and crystals that can help you achieve noticeable results in just two to three uses. Apply to clean, wet skin in a gentle, circular motion.
d) Relastyl™ Deep and Fine Line Repair or Perfect Rx Nite Serum are very popular as they both contain Matrixyl which can help diminish fine lines and wrinkles by stimulating hyaluronic

acid over 200% and collagen over 300%. Both hyaluronic acid and collagen production diminish as we age, causing sagging and wrinkled skin. Matrixyl is clinically proven to outperform retinol.

2. Emu oil and Hyaluronic Acid Cream or serum can also help hydrate fine lines around the mouth. Combine emu oil with face creams and apply to lined areas or wear it by itself. Emu oil does not clog pores.

3. Antioxidant-rich creams or serums can also help nourish and repair fine lines and wrinkles as well as protect face from further UV damage. Aging Eraser, High Potency Vitamin C Ester Serum or DMAE/C-Ester/ALA Retexturizing Creme can help repair and prevent lines and wrinkles.

4. To prevent lipstick from bleeding into fine lines around the mouth apply a lip fixative or lip liner before lipstick.

BEST BEAUTY BUYS FOR SMOOTHING LINES AROUND THE MOUTH

Exfoliants:
(To order visit www.hollywoodbeautysecrets.com)
• Microdermabrasion Scrub

Wrinkle Smoothers
(To order visit www.hollywoodbeautysecrets.com)
• Relastyl™ Deep and Fine Line Repair
• Perfect RX Nite Serum

Antioxidant-Rich Creams and Serum:
(To order visit www.hollywoodbeautysecrets.com)
• DMAE/ C-Ester/Alpha Lipoic Acid Retexurizing Creme

Part Five

- Aging Eraser™ by Age Advantage (Kinetin)
- High Potency Vitamin C Ester Serum™
- Hyaluronic Day & Nite Cream by derma e

Other Products Recommended:

(Available at your local health food store)
- Emu Oil
- DMAE Serum by Source Naturals

(Available at your local beauty supply store)
- CSI Sealed With a Kiss Lip Fixative

• **TIPS FOR BEAUTIFUL LIPS**

1. For a smooth lipstick base apply a wax-based lip balm like Chapstick (TM) before lipstick.

2. For fuller lips, use lip gloss in neutral or light colors such as flesh, nude or light berry. Avoid dark colors or lining lips. Both make lips appear smaller.

3. Here's an effective lip plumping recipe. NOTE: Do not try this if you have chapped or cracked lips. Combine 1 tbsp. mashed mango, ½ tsp. fresh lemon juice and a dash of cayenne pepper. Mash together and apply to lips for 2 minutes, then rinse. Products that contain enzymes can help plump up lips.

4. You'll find several lip-plumping products on the market, however many contain chemical ingredients. Lipworks is a doctor-formulated plumper that is made with 99% natural ingredients. It can help plump lips in just seven to 10 days. Tastes like tangerine too.

5. If you have full lips, enhance them with matte lipstick shades or apply a tinted gloss without lip liner.

6. To prevent lipstick from bleeding into fine lines around the mouth use a lip fixative as a base coat.

7. For uneven lips you'll need a flesh or nude colored lip liner to draw a very soft line outside of the thinner part of the lip. Color in the remainder of the lips with lip liner. Apply lip gloss. You may consider permanent make-up to remedy uneven lips. Read more about permanent make-up in "Anti-Aging Alternatives" in part twelve.

8. For longer lasting lipstick, choose a shade that closely matches your liner. Fill in entire lip area with lipliner, then apply lipstick and blot lips. Apply another coat of lipstick and blot again.

9. To keep lipstick from getting onto front teeth apply lipstick then suck and pull your thumb out of your mouth simultaneously. Excess lipstick will be on your thumb - not on teeth.

10. To soften lip color apply petroleum jelly or Vitamin E on lips after applying lipstick. Lip gloss creates softer, fuller looking lips.

11. To highlight lips for evening apply and blot lipstick twice. Then apply a pea-sized dab of frosted or gold lipstick in the center of the bottom lip.

12. Nude or flesh colored lip liner and a matching lipstick are lip essentials. Never wear lip liner that's darker than lipstick color. That's a very dated and unnatural look.

13. Choose lip gloss in flesh, nude or berry tones for a fresh look. Lawrence G, make-up artist to the stars, developed a beautiful line of lips glosses called S.w.e.e.t. Lacquer ™. Delicious tasting too.

14. Avoid orange lipstick as it makes teeth look yellow. Instead wear copper, coral or light peach. Red, wine, rose and raspberry shades make teeth look whitest.

BEST BEAUTY BUYS FOR BEAUTIFUL LIPS

Lip Smoothers:
(To order visit www.hollywoodbeautysecrets.com)
• Egyptian Magic All-Purpose Healer

(Available at your local drug store)
• Chapstick ®
• Blistex ® Revitalizer with AHA & Vitamin E
• Buzz Lip Honey

Lip Plumper:
(To order visit www.hollywoodbeautysecrets.com)
• LipWorks Lip Plumper

Glosses and Lipsticks:
(Available at your local drug store)
• Sally Hansen® Lip Quencher Daily Lip Moisturizer (Clear Nude, Clear Buff, Clear Mauve)
• Cover Girl® Lipslicks
• Almay® Pure Tints Protective Lip Care SPF 25

Other Products Recommended:
(Available at your local beauty Supply Shop)
* CSI Sealed With A Kiss (lip fixative)
* S.w.e.e.t. Lacquer ™ Lip Gloss by Lawrence G. To order contact 310-645-6454

● RELIEVING & PREVENTING COLD SORES

One of the best ways to prevent an outbreak of Herpes I and II is to avoid stress, which weakens the immune system. The following remedies have been know help prevent or bring relief to an outbreak. Check with your doctor before taking supplements.

1. Dr. Schulze Echinacea Plus formula for four to six weeks (2 drops, 4 times daily) is known to help prevent an outbreak both Herpes I and Herpes II. You can do this protocol two to three times a year.

2. Garlic or odorless (Kyolic) garlic capsules or tablets contain over 200 disease-fighting compounds which can help prevent certain viruses, infections, colds, flu, Herpes I and Herpes II and can fight bacteria, parasites, yeast overgrowth and fungus. Garlic has no known side effects and is safe to use on a long-term basis. Check with your doctor before taking supplements.

3. If you feel stressed or anxious, an outbreak may occur. Rescue Remedy, an oral spray can provide quick relief of stress or anxiety attacks.

4. Maintain a balanced pH. Diet influences pH. The more acidic the pH, the higher chance of having an outbreak. Eat fresh, raw

green leafy vegetables and salads, legumes, potatoes, fresh vegetable juices, whole grains and fruits including citrus. Avoid refined and processed foods such as white flour products, rice, crackers, cakes, cookies, corn syrup, dairy products, all meats including hot dogs, sausage, cold cuts, burgers, fish, shellfish, chicken, vinegar, ketchup, mayonnaise, pickles, spicy foods, hot sauce, saturated fats, hydrogenated oils, margarine, alcohol, soft drinks, juices, black tea and coffee. There are many books available in health food stores that address balancing your pH.

5. The moment you feel an outbreak coming on, taking Lysine, red marine algae or olive leaf extract can help prevent the outbreak. Red marine algae oxygenates the body and supports the immune system. Olive leaf extract contains anti-viral, anti-fungal and antibacterial agents. Taking Kyolic (odorless) garlic caps can help eliminate many viruses, including the Herpes I and II virus.

6. During an outbreak of herpes the following remedies have been known to help provide relief. Check with your physician.

a) Thorne Glycgel contains licorice root, L-Lysine and zinc which are known to help heal sores quickly.
b) Applying a tincture of calendula can help relieve sores.
c) Antioxidants such as Vitamins A, C, E and grape seed can be beneficial.
d) Red marine algae provides immune support.
e) Applying a cotton ball soaked in Vitamin O or H-Balm can help relieve discomfort and speed heal sores.
f) Bromelain and digestive enzymes such as Vitalzymes ® have been known to help destroy the protein coat of the herpes virus.
g) Taking cimetidine, the active ingredient in some over-the-counter antacids, during an outbreak can help reduce the

number and duration of future outbreaks. Check with your doctor for dosage.

h) Ozonated olive oil or an ozone sauna are also known to help provide relief of herpes.

BEST BEAUTY BUYS FOR COLD SORES/HERPES

(To order call 1-800-HERBDOC)
- Dr. Schultz Echinacea Plus

(Available at your local health food store)
- Lysine Liquid Extract
- Red Marine Algae
- Rescue Remedy by Bach (oral spray)
- Olive Leaf
- Vitamin O
- H-Balm
- Calendula

(Available at your local drug store)
- Cimetidine (antacid ingredient).

• REMEDIES FOR CANKER SORES

1. Yogurt can help bring relief to canker sores. Eat yogurt regularly or take acidophilus tablets on an empty stomach. Swish plain yogurt in your mouth in the area of the canker sore for a minute or two. Then swallow or spit out. Do not rinse mouth.

2. Avoid spicy and acidic foods such as tomatoes and citrus fruits.

3. Dab the canker sore with a black tea bag. Tannins in tea can help reduce inflammation.

4. Reduce stress. Rescue Remedy oral spray can help calm you during stressful times.

5. Kanka by Blistex® can help.

BEST BEAUTY BUYS FOR RELIEVING CANKER SORES

(Available at your local health food store)
- Acidophilus
- Plain Yogurt
- Rescue Remedy by Bach

(Available at your local drug store)
- Kanka by Blistex®

• ELIMINATING LIP HAIR

Menstruation and hormone changes can cause facial hair to darken and become more noticeable. Waxing removes natural peach fuzz, can cause ingrown hairs and can often clog pores. Instead of waxing consider bleaching lip hair using a gentle facial bleaching agent. Then use cuticle scissors and a magnifying mirror to carefully clip long lip hair. Forget the myth that lip hair will grow back thicker and darker if clipped. During my modeling career, I've done many of close-up lip shots and this is the technique I use to keep lip hair out of sight.

BEST BEAUTY BUYS FOR ELIMINATING LIP HAIR

(Available at your local health food store)
- Jolen ™ Crème Bleach
- Cuticle Scissors

• REMEDIES FOR WHITER TEETH
A winning smile gives a positive first impression. Yellow teeth can be a sign of aging. To keep your pearlies white and your age a secret here are some effective remedies:

1. Yellow teeth can be easily whitened by regular brushing with toothpaste that contains peroxide and whiteners.

2. Combine a mixture of one part hydrogen peroxide and one part distilled or bottled water in a small sterilized glass or plastic bottle. After drinking tea, cola, coffee or wine, simply swish the mixture through your teeth like mouthwash for one minute. Spit out mixture then rinse with water. Your teeth will be instantly whiter.

3. Dip your toothbrush in hydrogen peroxide and baking soda then gently brush teeth.

4. Strawberries can help fade coffee, tea and cola stains. Bite into a strawberry and rub it over teeth.

5. Forget whitening wands. Whitening strips are much more effective, reasonably priced and can quickly and safely whiten teeth. The strips help the peroxide gel remain on the teeth.

6. For more serious yellowing, consider laser bleaching which can instantly remedy yellow teeth. Results are quick, but instant gratification is expensive. Prices vary from $400 or more. Gums are protected by applying a wax coating before the peroxide and laser. The procedure may cause discomfort. Pain relievers, such as Tylenol ™ should minimize throbbing. Ask for a fluoride treatment after the procedure to prevent tooth sensitivity. Once you've made this investment, you'll need to maintain the whiteness so be sure to invest in either a custom bleaching kit or simply use whitening strips regularly.

BEST BEAUTY BUYS FOR WHITER TEETH

(Available at your local drug store)
- Supersmile® Toothpaste (helps whiten, removes stains, plaque and protects enamel from becoming stained)
- Prevident 5000 Plus (fluoride treatment)

Whitening Strips & Trays:
(Available at your local drug store)
- Crest® Whitestrips
- Rembrandt's® Superior Whitening Toothpaste and Trays

• VENEERS FOR TEETH
For gaps, thin, crooked or chipped teeth consider veneers. There are two types of veneers: plastic (less expensive) or porcelain (more expensive, easier to maintain and last longer). Both use resin and a high-intensity beam to bond to teeth. Before application, a layer of the tooth's surface is removed. Be sure to research dentists who specialize in veneers as the procedure is costly and requires dental expertise.

Lip & Oral Care

• BONDING TEETH
Bonding works well for filling in small chips. Most dentists offer bonding. It is often covered by dental insurance. The procedure is quick and painless.

• GRINDING YOUR TEETH
Many Americans (80% of the population) grind their teeth while sleeping. A night guard merely cushions the back teeth but does not relieve you of grinding. You can still get cracks in your teeth and experience a tired jaw from the pressure of grinding on a night guard. So I did some investigating and discovered an interesting alternative. Rather than investing in a night guard, consider a TMJ appliance. Your family dentist can have one made for you. The appliance simply clips to the front of the teeth, preventing your back teeth from grinding together. I no longer wake up with a sore jaw and my bite has not been effected whatsoever. This appliance costs about half the price of a night guard!

• RELIEVING A TOOTHACHE
Apply a temporary obtundant dressing until you can see a dentist. Obtundant dressings like clove oil work by irritating the surface of the skin and react with the body's natural endorphins (feel-good transmitters) to ease toothache pain. Try either of these:

1. Apply clove oil to gauze. Place saturated gauze on throbbing tooth.

2. Apply toothache gel which you can find in a drug store.

BEST BEAUTY BUYS FOR RELIEVING A TOOTHACHE

(Available at your local health food store)
- Clove Oil

Nail, Hand & Foot Care

- **RECOGNIZING NAIL DISORDERS**
Lack of certain vitamins or nutrients, dark nail polish colors, allergies, drug reactions, smoking, lupus, thyroid problems, liver or kidney disease, psoriasis, eczema or warts can effect nail color and texture. See a physician to discuss treatment.

1. Pale nails may indicate anemia. You may need more iron. See "Food Fixes for Nails" in this section.

2. Grey or Beige Nails may be a result of taking antibiotics or that you may need more Vitamin B12. See "Food Fixes for Nails".

3. Yellow Nails may be a result of wearing dark polish, not wearing base coat, smoking or applying self-tanning creams and hair products that stain. Lung disease may also cause yellow nails.

4. Nail breakage and peeling or brittle nails may be an indication that you are low in any one of the following: iron, essential fatty acids, calcium, zinc, protein, biotin, Vitamin A, B6 or B12. See "Food Fixes for Nails". Brittle nails may also be a sign of poor digestion or that you may need to condition nails. Always wear rubber gloves when doing housework, using detergents, chemicals, or disinfecting wipes. At night massage nails using olive, castor, coconut or almond oil, Vitamin A or E, and top with a generous portion of petroleum jelly. Wear cotton gloves to keep in moisture. To strengthen nails, apply protein formula daily for two to three weeks.

5. A sign of nail fungus is indicated by a gray or brown colored nail. Apply a topical anti-fungal product to affected nail daily or try the natural nail soak recipe below. Be patient. Fungus can take several months to remedy. For mild cases of fungus applying tea tree oil, grapefruit seed extract or citrus-based topical anti-fungal products can help. Oral anti-fungal medications should be used as a last resort as they can be extremely hard on the liver, and you will require doctor's supervision. Consider this natural anti-fungal soak recipe: You'll need 6 ounces of fresh ginger and 4 to 5 pieces of Chinese licorice root. Chinese licorice root is more potent than the America version. Find Chinese licorice root at the health food store or an Asian market. Ginger is available in all grocery stores. Using your mallet, mash the licorice root and ginger, then place into a pot of 4 to 5 cups of water. Bring to a boil for 5 to 7 minutes. Let cool slightly, then strain. Dip fingers or feet in the warm tea-colored water for 15 to 20 minutes. Then towel dry.

6. Pitted or bumpy nails may be caused by eczema, warts or psoriasis. Your doctor may recommend a steroid cream or injection. Use ridge filling base coat to create smooth looking nails. Apply Vitamin A and E oil to nail beds frequently.

7. Thin, weak nails can be strengthened using protein nail hardener. Biotin supplements and biotin-rich foods increase the thickness of nails. See "Food Fixes for Nails".

8. Ridges are a sign of normal aging or can be an indication of poor absorption of vitamins and minerals. Use a ridge filling base coat to create smooth looking nails.

9. Pink or white areas on nails are due to trauma or you may

need more zinc in your diet. Did you bump your finger? This could also be a sign of an underlying kidney problem.

10. Taking silica gel along with prenatal vitamins is known to help quickly grow strong, long nails and also helps speed hair growth.

BEST BEAUTY BUYS FOR NAIL DISORDERS

Nail Strengtheners:
(Available at your local beauty supply store)
- Nailtiques® Formula 2 **PLUS** (protein formula for peeling, splitting nails)
- Nailtiques® Formula 2 (protein nail hardener for thin, weak nails)
- Qtica™Natural Nail Growth Stimulator

Basecoats:
(You may use nail strengthener as a basecoat.)
(Available at your local beauty supply store)
- NailTek™Foundation Formula (base coat, ridge filler, nail strengthener, prevents yellow nails, smoothes pitted or bumpy nails)
- Orly Bonder (rubberized formulation ensures a lasting manicure)

(Available at your local health food store)
Other Products Recommended:
- Almond or Olive Oil
- Castor Oil
- Coconut Oil
- Lanolin (don't use if you're allergic to wool)

- Silica Gel

Anti-fungals:
(Available at your local health food store)
- Tea Tree oil
- NutriBiotic GSE Liquid Concentrate Grapefruit Seed Extract
- Chinese Licorice Root
(Available at your local beauty supply store)
- Varisi By Alva Jade (organic citrus anti-fungal)
(Available at www.hollywoodbeautysecrets.com)
- Vitamin A and E Wrinkle Treatment Oil

• FOOD FIXES FOR NAILS
Proper nutrition can strengthen and smooth nails. Eat a diet rich in calcium, biotin, protein, iron, Beta Carotene, Vitamins A, B, C, E, and zinc. Include a variety of yellow, orange, and red fruits, vegetables, grains, leafy greens, raw nuts and healthy oils in your diet. Here are some beneficial foods for nails:
- Beta carotene-rich foods include carrots, tomatoes, watermelon, sweet potatoes, papaya, broccoli, spinach and green leafy vegetables.
- Vitamin A-rich foods include egg yolks, oysters and non-fat milk.
- Vitamin B-rich foods include red meat, turkey, chicken, butter, eggs, peanut butter, bananas, whole grains, fish, milk, cheese and yogurt.
- Vitamin C-rich foods include cantaloupe, strawberries, tomatoes, red peppers, citrus fruits and green peas.

- Vitamin E-rich foods include salmon, lean meats, almonds, leafy greens, olives, olive and sesame oil, legumes and Vitamin E supplements.
- Calcium-rich foods include low-fat cheese and milk, butter, tofu, sesame seeds, sardines, dark leafy vegetables, carrots and fresh carrot juice. Take calcium supplements daily.
- Protein-rich foods include eggs, chicken, turkey, quail, lamb, red meat, liver, fish (including sardines), whey or soy protein powder and beans.
- Biotin-rich foods include cereals, milk, egg yolks, peanut butter, lentils and cauliflower. Biotin supplements are recommended.
- Zinc-rich foods include eggs, liver and milk. Take zinc supplements daily.
- Iron-rich foods include liver, spinach and dark leafy greens.
- Healthy nuts, seeds include almonds, walnuts, flax, sunflower and pumpkin seeds. Healthy oils include grape seed, flax seed oil, olive, sesame and almond oils, avocados and EFA.S (Essential Fatty Acids).
- Silicia gel can help nails grow quickly as well as help speed hair growth.

- **BRIGHTENING YELLOW OR STAINED NAILS**

If you have yellow or stained nails the following nail brightening remedies can help. Do not use more than one remedy at a time or you may risk splitting or drying out nails. After each remedy moisturize nails with shea butter, olive, coconut or almond oil and top with petroleum jelly. Wear gloves. Wait 24 to 48 hours before applying polish.

1. An effective and affordable way to remove yellow stains from nails is with baking soda and lemon juice. Combine 1 tbsp.

lemon juice with 1 to 2 tbsp. baking soda to make a paste. Wet hands and rub nails with the paste-like exfoliator. Leave on nails for five minutes. Then rinse. If you have pigmentation spots on your hands you may want to use this paste as an exfoliator and spot fader, or simply scrub hands nightly with baking soda.

2. Very light buffing removes yellow stains from nails. Use the smoothest grit of a 4-way buffing block or file. Rinse with water. Apply olive oil or Vitamin A and E oil to moisturize nails.

3. Apply alpha hydroxy acid (AHA) cream on hands and nails two to three nights a week. AHA and can help remove stains from nails and exfoliates skin.

4. Apply whitening toothpaste on an extra soft toothbrush. Scrub nails gently for one minute. Rinse with soapy water.

5. Dip hands and nails in soy yogurt. Soy contains natural bleaching agents. Add a squirt of lemon for extra stubborn stains. Allow yogurt to dry for 10 to 15minutes. Rinse with soapy water.

6. Apply base coat before applying polish. Base coat can help prevent yellow stains and makes a perfect ridge filler for smooth polish application. Wearing dark nail polish can stain nails. Stick to lighter colors.

7. FluorX® Stop Yellow is a hydrogen peroxide gel. Apply gel to nails for two to three minutes. Rinse with soapy water

8. For a quick fix, use Yello-Out™Clear Acrylic Top Coat as

a base coat. Its bluish hue provides a temporary fix that brightens nails instantly. Apply quick-dry top coat or nail color over Yello-Out™ to seal in brightness.

BEST BEAUTY BUYS FOR BRIGHTENING STAINED NAILS

Nail Brighteners:
(Available at your local drug store)
- FluorX® Stop Yellow
- Yello-Out™ Clear Acrylic Top Coat (bluish hue)

Base Coats:
(Available at your local beauty supply shop)
- Nail Tek™ Foundation (strengthens, smoothes ridges and prevents yellowing)
- Orly® Bonder (rubberized base coat ensures lasting polish and prevents yellowing)
- Creative Nail, Stickey Base coat (rubberized)

Other Products Recommended:
(Available at your local beauty supply shop)
- 4-Way Buffers and Files

• REJUVENATING HAND SECRETS
We use our hands for so many activities: housework, dishes, cooking, sports, gardening and caring for our family and pets. Hands don't have many oil glands so they can quickly look aged - even in our 20's! To keep hands looking youthful, try these quick and effective rejuvenating secrets:

1. Keep hands out of the sun. Sun damage can begin within 60 seconds of exposure. Without protection you may experience age spots on your hands by the time you reach your 40's. It's not age, but sun that's causing these spots. When spending time outdoors, be sure to wear cotton gloves to protect hands from damaging rays. Wear gloves when you're driving as UV rays penetrate windshield glass. Keep a pair of gloves in the car or in your purse. Wear sunscreen on hands whenever possible.

2. Water is very damaging to hands and nails. It's the number one cause of splitting, peeling nails as well as stripping moisture from hands. When hands are frequently in water (washing dishes, doing housework, cooking) you may also risk developing arthritis in your hands. Wear rubber gloves to protect against dry hands, brittle, peeling nails and arthritis. Before starting your chores, apply hand lotion or olive, coconut or almond oil onto hands, put on some cotton gloves and wear rubber gloves over top. When your work is done, you'll be rewarded with soft hands and healthy nails!

3. A Hollywood manicurist shared this interesting tip with me. Don't soak nails in water to soften cuticles. As mentioned above, water causes splitting, peeling nails. Let your manicurist know that you prefer she massage oil into your nails and cuticles. Bring your own olive or coconut oil with you when you visit your manicurist. Once cuticles have been massaged with oil, push cuticles back. Do not cut cuticles. Cuticles protect nails from infection.

4. Frequently apply antioxidant-rich lotion, oil or serum to hands. Keep lotion in every room in the house so you'll be reminded to moisturize. Keep hand lotion in your purse.

5. To keep hands looking youthful, exfoliate them regularly.
Below are some very effective choices for exfoliating:
a) Apply creams or serums that contain antioxidant-rich
ingredients such as alpha lipoic acid, retinoids (Vitamin A),
AHA's, C-Ester, Vitamin E, Green Tea, or Matrixyl. Apply
before bed.
b) Milk is a handy exfoliator too. Warm a bowl of milk in the
microwave for 15 to 20 seconds. Massage olive, coconut,
Vitamin A or E oil into nails and cuticles. Turn hands, palms up,
and dip them for 10 to 15 minutes while keeping nails out of the
milk. Remember that soaking nails can cause peeling and
splitting. The lactic acid in milk exfoliates skin and helps fade
pigmentation spots. The fat in milk also softens and moisturizes
skin.
c) While in the shower or when washing up before bed, exfoliate
hands with baking soda. Gently scrub wet hands using a handful
of baking soda to remove dry skin, diminish wrinkled knuckles
and prevent future age spots. Follow with one of the creams in
the Best Beauty Buys section or use your own personal favorite.
d) Papaya is a great exfoliant for hands and cuticles. Combine 1
tbsp. mashed papaya with 1 tbsp. olive oil and massage into
hands and cuticles. Apply produce bags on hands. Wait 10
minutes, then remove bags. Rinse hands and push cuticles back
using your thumb nails or an orange wood stick. Apply
moisturizer.
e) Yogurt and lemon juice can help fade pigmentation spots on
hands and arms. Mix two tablespoons yogurt with a squirt of
lemon juice. Apply and let dry. Then rinse.

6. To diminish wrinkled knuckles, buff them lightly using the
finest grit of a 4-way buffing block. Then apply antioxidant-rich
cream such as Relastyl™ or Perfect RX Night Serum. Both

contain Matrixyl to help stimulate collagen over 300% and hyaluronic production over 200%. These products can help diminish age spots and help firm and hydrate the hands and knuckles. Use serum nightly on extremely dry or mature hands. Follow with shea butter, coconut or castor oil or petroleum jelly and wear cotton gloves.

7. Fade age spots and rejuvenate hands with L.E.D. Therapy. L.E.D. Therapy can help diminish age spots and has many other anti-aging benefits. For example, if you suffer from sore joints or arthritis in your hands L.E.D. therapy can help relieve pain. It stimulates collagen production which can help prevent wrinkled knuckles, diminish age spots, tighten and firm sagging skin and more. It's safe to use on any color or age skin! See more information about anti-aging L.E.D. Therapy in "Affordable Ways to Look 10 or More Years Younger", at the beginning of this book. A home unit is also now available. For more information contact louisa@hollywoodbeautysecrets.com.

8. Buff nails regularly with a soft chamois nail buffer. Buffing can help strengthen and stimulate nail growth.

9. Carrying heavy items like grocery bags or boxes creates blood flow to the veins in the hands. This increase in blood causes the veins to protrude or enlarge. Veiny hands are associated with aged-looking hands. Whenever possible use a shopping cart or a dolly to transport groceries, boxes or heavy bags. When veins are prominent on hands they can be rejuvenated with Sclerotherapy or fat injections. See an experienced phlebologist (vein specialist). Find resources for vein specialists and practioners who do fat injections in "Anti-Aging Alternatives".

10. A top hand model from New York shared this rejuvenating tip with me. He applies Chaptick® to his knuckles and cuticles so they appear more youthful in front of the camera. It immediately diminishes dry cuticles and helps smooth knuckles.

BEST BEAUTY BUYS FOR REJUVENATING HANDS

Hand Cream and Oil Suggestions:

(To order visit www.hollywoodbeautysecrets.com)
- Relastyl™ Deep & Fine Line Repair
- Perfect RX Nite Serum
- Hand Crème Age Reversal Formula by derma e
- DMAE/Alpha Lipoic/C-Ester Retexturizing Ceme
- High Potency Vitamin C-Ester Serum™ by Age Advantage
- Hyaluronic Acid Firming Serum by Derma e
- Vitamin A and E Wrinkle Treatment Oil

(Available at your local drug store)
- Aquaphor® Healing Ointment for Dry, Cracked skin
- Sally Hansen® 18 Hour Protection Hand Crème
- Vaseline® Dual Action Hydroxy Formula
- St. Ives® Swiss Vanilla with Vitamin E for Dry Skin

Nail Hardeners:
(Available at your local Beauty Supply Shop)
- Nailtiques® Formula 2 PLUS (protein for peeling, splitting nails)
- Nailtiques® Formula 2 (protein nail hardener for thin, weak nails)
- Qtica™ Natural Nail Growth Stimulator

Other Products Recommended:
(Available at your local drug store or beauty supply shop)
- 4-Way buffing block and files
- Cotton Gloves
- Nail Buffer
- Chapstick®
- Coconut Oil

(To order visit www.hollywoodbeautysecrets.com)
- Light Therapy Unit

• SOLVING COMMON NAIL PROBLEMS

1. To prevent nail polish from chipping or peeling, apply one thin coat of base coat and two thin coats of nail polish. Finish with one thin coat of quick-dry top coat. NOTE: Thin coats of polish provide a longer lasting manicure. Thick coats of polish peel off within a day or two.

2. For a longer lasting manicure, apply a thin coat of quick-dry top coat every two days.

3. To prevent bubbles in polish, dry nails thoroughly after washing. Before applying polish wipe nails using Isopropyl alcohol with a cotton pad to remove residual oil left from soap or moisturizer. Instead of shaking the polish bottle, try rolling it in your palms.

4. For weak nails, or those that grow slowly, consider taking silica gel which is known to help strengthen nails and speed growth. Prenatal vitamins can also speed nail growth.

5. To prevent splitting, peeling nails keep hands out of water and ALWAYS wear rubber gloves when handling cleanser, detergent, antibacterial wipes, doing housework, laundry or washing produce. For dry or peeling nails, apply protein nail hardener daily for three weeks. It dries in about two minutes so be sure to apply it daily. Your nails will be strong and split-free. NOTE: Many individuals are known to have a latex allergy. Vinyl gloves are available at your local drug store.

BEST BEAUTY BUYS FOR COMMON NAIL PROBLEMS

Quick-Dry Top Coats:
(Available at your local beauty supply shop)
• Orly® In a Snap Nail Finish
• Sally Hansen® Dries Instantly Top Coat

Nail Hardeners:
(Available at your local beauty supply shop)
• Nailtiques® Formula 2 PLUS (protein for peeling, splitting nails)
• Nailtiques® Formula 2 (protein nail hardener for thin, weak nails)
• Essie Millionails Nail Strengthener
• Q-Tica™ Natural Nail Growth Stimulator
(Available at your local health food store)
• Silica Gel
• Prenatal Vitamins

• **LOUISA'S 5-STEP MANICURE**
As a top hands and parts model the ability to do my own manicure saves a production time and money. Directors,

producers and photographers can always rely on me to arrive on set with my hands looking picture perfect. Here's what you'll need to do my simple 5-step manicure: acetone-free polish remover, a bowl of warm milk, almond or olive oil, an orange wood stick, a 4-way nail file, a padded buffing block, 70% isopropyl alcohol, cotton pads, base coat, nail polish and quick-dry top coat.

1. Remove nail polish with acetone-free polish remover.

2. To rejuvenate hands and diminish wrinkled knuckles, warm a bowl of milk in the microwave (about 15 to 20 seconds, or until warm - not hot). Apply olive oil to nails and soak hands palms up keeping nails out of the milk. Rinse after 10 minutes. If you don't have time to soak in milk simply use the finest grit of a 4-way nail buffing block to gently buff wrinkled knuckles. Then rinse hands.

3. Massage olive oil into hands and on nails for one to two minutes. Push cuticles back using your thumb nails or an orange wood stick wrapped in cotton. NEVER cut cuticles as they protect nails from infection.

4. File nails using a 4-way nail file (use medium grit). File very gently, using a back and forth motion. Yes, back and forth, top nail experts agree with me. Nail experts agree with me. Shape nails using the medium grit and lightly buff nail tops smooth, using the finest grit of the 4-way nail file or use a chamois buffer.

5. Wipe nails with 70% isopropyl alcohol, using a cotton pad. Alcohol removes traces of oil or soap. This prevents bubbles and allows polish to better adhere. Apply one thin coat of base coat. Let dry. Then apply two thin coats of nail polish. Let dry.

Finish with one thin coat of quick- dry top coat. *NOTE:* Applying thin coats of polish prevents peeling and ensures a lasting manicure. After polish dries apply Relastyl™ or one of the suggestions in the Best Beauty Buys that follow.

BEST BEAUTY BUYS FOR LOUISA'S MANICURE

Polish Remover:
- Mary Ann B. Nail Laquer Remover (To order email Cheryl at cf2000@comcast.net Mention this book to receive a 10% discount.)

Other Products Recommended:
(Available at your local drug store)
- 4-Way Buffing Blocks and Files
- Orange Wood Sticks
- Isopropyl Alcohol

Base Coats:
(Available at your local beauty supply shop)
- Orly® Oil-Free Nail Polish Remover
- Nailteck ™ Foundation Base Coat (strengthens, prevents yellow stains and smoothes nails)
- Orly® Bonder (rubberized)

Popular Nail Polish Colors:
(Available at your local beauty supply shop)
- Essie - Ballet Slippers, Curtain Call, Dune Road (various light pink colors)
- Orly ® Who's Who Pink (many celebrities wear this opalized pink color), Sheer Buff (light beige color)

- OPI - Coney Island Cotton Candy (fleshy pink color), Sweetheart (baby pink color), Malaysian Myst (nude color)

(Available at your local drug store)
- Revlon® Sheer Flicker (baby pink color)
- Maybelline ® Express Finish; Barely Pink (light baby pink color)
- Revlon® makes long-lasting nail color in many shades

Quick-Dry Top Coats:
(Available at your local drug store)
- Orly® Sec'n Dry
- Sally Hansen® Dries Instantly Top Coat

Wrinkle Diminishers & Collagen Stimulators:
(To order visit www.hollywoodbeautysecrets.com)
- Relastyl™ Deep and Fine Line Wrinkle Repair
- Perfect RX Nite Serum
- High Potency Vitamin C-Ester Serum

- **LOUISA'S 30-MINUTE PEDICURE**
You can do this quick, effective pedicure at home in under 30 minutes. This is what you'll need: one quart homogenized milk, a pumice stone or foot file, an orange wood stick, a 4-way nail file, a set of toe separators or two tissues, base coat, quick-dry nail polish, moisturizing lotion, 70% isopropyl alcohol, and a foot bath or large plastic tub for soaking feet.

1. Remove polish using acetone-free nail polish remover.

2. Pour milk into a large bowl and microwave for two to three minutes. Milk should be warm to hot – not boiling hot.

Microwave using 15-second increments until milk is correct temperature then pour into footbath. Add an equal amount of warm water. Soak feet for 10 minutes. The lactic acid in milk softens cuticles and exfoliates dry, dead skin. The fat in milk moisturizes skin.

3. After soaking, buff callused heels and bottoms of toes using a pumice stone or foot file. Use an orange wood stick wrapped in cotton to push back softened cuticles. Never cut cuticles as they protect nails from infection.

4. Use the finest grit of a 4-way file to smooth and buff tops of nails. Trim toe nails straight across in a square shape. Do not trim nails too short. Rinse feet with tepid water. Then towel dry.

5. Place toenail separators between toes or twist a tissue and weave it between toes. Use a cotton pad to wipe nails with isopropyl alcohol. This removes all traces of milk fat or oils which prevents bubbles and allows polish to adhere better.

6. Apply one thin coat of base coat and two thin coats of quick-dry nail polish. Thin coats of polish are less likely to peel off than thick coats ensuring a lasting pedicure. Quick-dry polish takes only 10 minutes to dry to a hard finish. Then apply moisturizing lotion.

BEST BEAUTY BUYS FOR LOUISA'S PEDICURE

Polish Remover:
• Mary Ann B. Nail Laquer Remover. To order email Cheryl at cf2000@comcast.net. Mention this book to receive a 10% discount.

(Available at your local beauty supply shop)
- Orly ® Oil-Free Nail Polish Remover

Other Products Recommended:
(Available at your local drug store)
- 4-Way Buffing Blocks and Files
- Orangewood Sticks
- Isopropyl Alcohol
- Foot Bath
- Foot File
- Toe Nail Separators

Base Coats:
- Nailteck™ Foundation Base Coat (strengthens, prevents yellow stains and smoothes nails)
- Creative Nail Design, Stickey Base Coat
- Orly® Bonder (rubberized)

Quick-Dry Polishes:
- Revlon® Top Speed (comes in a variety of shades)
- Maybelline® Express Finish (comes in a variety of shades)

Foot Creams and Oils:
(To order visit www.hollywoodbeautysecrets.com)
- Luxuriant Cracked Heel Relief™
- Egyptian Magic All-Purpose Healing Cream
- Vitamin A and E Wrinkle Treatment Oil

(Available at your local drug store)
- Herbacin™ Kamille and Glycerine Cream
- Aquaphor® Healing Ointment (for dry, cracked skin)

- Vaseline® Dual Action Hydroxy Formula

- **AVOIDING & RELIEVING INGROWN TOENAILS**
To *avoid* ingrown toenails follow these easy steps:
1. Trim toe nails straight across in a square shape.

2. Never trim toe nails short. Instead, keep them medium in length and trim them more often.

3. Avoid shoes that are too small as they pinch and put pressure on toenails.

To *relieve* an ingrown toe nail:
1. Fill a foot bath with warm water and 1/4 cup Morton Salts or sea salt. Soak feet for 10 minutes then rinse feet with tepid water. Dry feet thoroughly.

2. Wedge a small piece of cotton under the corner of the ingrown nail. Do this nightly for two to three weeks.

3. If you experience oozing or pain see a podiatrist.

BEST BEAUTY BUYS FOR INGROWN TOENAILS

(Available at your local drug store)
- Morton Salts
- Sea Salt

Part Six

• RELIEVING CRACKED, DRY HEELS & FEET

1. For quick relief of dry heels and feet, try Luxuriant Cracked Heel Relief™ as it saturates the skin to help heal deep cracks and chronic rough, dry heels. It contains more than 10 essential oils.

2. Another great choice is Egyptian Magic All-Purpose Healing Cream. It's an amazing balm that's loaded with bees wax, honey, bee propollis, olive oil and natural ingredients. A top seller.

3. Zim's Crack Crème™can help diminish cracks and dryness. Use it daily.

4. Apply products that contain urea, salicylic acid, Vitamin A, E or 10 to 20% alpha hyrdoxy acid to eliminate callus build-up and cracked heels. You can purchase 20% AHA from your dermatologists office and 10% AHA at a local drug store.

5. Walking around the house in bare feet can cause cracked heels. Moisturize feet regularly and wear socks whenever possible. Wearing mules, sandals and sling-back shoes can cause cracked heels. After wearing these types of shoes moisturize feet using the products in #7 and put on some socks. Try to wear socks with shoes whenever possible.

6. Use a pumice stone or foot file at least two to three times a week in the shower. Apply lotion after showering to seal in moisture.

7. For extra-dry feet, slather coconut oil, cocoa or shea butter on feet, top with petroleum jelly and put on a pair of socks. Leave on overnight.

8. Heat 1 tbsp. cocoa butter or coconut oil and add 2 drops peppermint essential oil. Apply mixture to feet then wrap in cellophane. Put on some socks. Wait 20 to 45 minutes then remove cellophane, massage feet and replace socks.

9. Here's a fantastic foot softener and dead skin eliminator. In a blender or food processor combine the pulp of ½ ripe papaya, 1 medium sized can of pineapple slices in natural juice, 3 tbsp. sea salt, 1 tbsp. cayenne pepper and 1 tbsp. white vinegar. Blend until smooth. Split the mixture into two plastic produce bags or two zip lock bags that are big enough to accommodate each foot. Place the bags in a foot bath or plastic tub. Then place each foot in each bag and wrap a small towel around each foot. Move your feet around and wriggle your toes in the bags to help eliminate dead skin. Rinse mixture off after 30 minutes.

10. Persistently cracked skin may indicate foot fungus or athlete's foot. Try the foot bath that follows until you can see your doctor.

BEST BEAUTY BUYS FOR RELIEVING CRACKED, DRY HEELS AND FEET

Cracked Heel Eliminators:
(To order visit www.hollywoodbeautysecrets.com)
- Luxuriant Cracked Heel Relief™
- Egyptian Magic All-Purpose Healing Cream
- Vitamin A and E Wrinkle Treatment Wrinkle

(Available at your local drug store)
- Zim's Crack Crème®
- Pumice Stone

- Foot File

- **RECIPES FOR ATHLETE'S FOOT**

Dry, callused feet can be a sign of athlete's foot. See your doctor or a podiatrist. Until doing so, try one of the following for temporary relief:

1. Cloves can help fight athlete's foot. Place 5 tbsp. cloves in an old clean cotton sock or in a piece of cheesecloth. Tie with string. Steep the clove bag in 3 cups boiling water for 10 minutes. Let sit until warm and pour clove water into foot bath. Soak feet for 20 minutes.

2. Combine 4 drops clove and 6 drops peppermint essential oils with 2 tbsp. almond oil. Rub mixture on feet. Put on some socks.

3. Athlete's foot cream can be found in your local drug store. It can help soften dry, cracked feet.

BEST BEAUTY BUYS FOR ATHLETE'S FOOT

(Available at your local health food store)
- Clove Essential Oil
- Peppermint Essential Oil

Leg & Body Care

• EFFECTIVE BODY SCRUBS

To keep body skin smooth and flawless, frequent exfoliating (sloughing off skin) is a must. Exfoliating the body boosts circulation of the blood and the lymphatic system, stimulates collagen and elastin production and helps tighten and smooth skin. Focus on tummy, buttocks, thighs and arms to prevent sagging skin. Moisturize skin after bathing to seal in moisture. Indulge in one of the following beneficial body scrubs two to three times a week.

1. Before bathing, exfoliate and smooth skin by dry brushing with a natural bristle body brush. Dry brushing stimulates collagen production, helps eliminate dead skin cells and helps clear the lymphatic system. Don't brush too hard. Skin should be pink when done correctly. Start at your ankles and brush up the thighs using a C-shaped motion. Brush toward the heart. Then start at the wrists and work up the arms. Include brushing your torso and buttocks.

2. In the shower, apply baking soda to a face cloth and gently rub the cloth over entire body in a circular motion. Rinse with tepid water. Your skin will feel like silk.

3. This scrub is easy to do and very effective. Mix 2 cups sea salt with ½ cup almond or olive oil. DO NOT apply on the facial area or on irritated, broken skin. Rub scrub on wet skin in a gentle, circular motion. Start at ankles and continue application up thighs. Then start at wrists continuing up arms and include the torso and buttocks. You may prefer to sit in a tub with a few

inches of tepid water while applying the salt scrub. Then rinse with tepid water.

4. Here's another easy moisturizing scrub. Mix 3/4 cup corn meal, 1/2 cup milk and 1/4 cup plain yogurt. Apply in a warm room. Stand in the shower or tub and rub the mixture onto the body, using a circular scrubbing motion. Rinse with tepid water. Finish with a cool rinse.

5. This exfoliating body mask gently removes dead skin cells and evens out skin tones. You'll need plain or soy yogurt. In a warm room, apply one to two cups plain yogurt on entire body including face. Wait 10 to 15 minutes until dry then rinse with tepid water.

6. For sensitive skin combine two cups warm, unsweetened apple sauce, 1/4 cup almond or olive oil, and 1 tbsp. lemon or orange juice. Stand in the shower or tub and apply mixture on body. Wait 10 minutes then rinse with tepid water.

7. For dry skin, mix 4 tbsp. almond or olive oil, 3 tbsp. lemon juice and 1 tbsp. honey. Stand in the shower or sit in a tub and massage onto dry skin. Rinse with tepid water.

8. Pumpkin removes impurities and heals skin. Mix one can of pumpkin with 3/4 cup plain yogurt and 3 tbsp. lemon or orange juice. In a warm room apply the mixture on entire body including face. Wait 10 to 15 minutes then rinse with tepid water.

9. Papaya is a natural alternative to Retin A. Cut 2 papayas in half and remove the pulp. Rub the inside of the papaya peels all over clean body, including face. The moist residue is loaded with exfoliating and brightening enzymes. You may prefer to buy only

one papaya and apply the mashed papaya pulp. It's up to you, however this is a little messier as the pulp will fall to the floor. You'll still be left with the enzyme-rich residue. Wait 10 minutes then rinse with tepid water. The enzymes in papaya exfoliate, brighten and remove impurities from skin.

10. If you have eczema, try this body mask or apply the mix to dry patches. Combine 1 mashed papaya with 1 cup plain yogurt. Apply to clean skin. Wait 10 minutes, then rinse with tepid water.

BEST BEAUTY BUYS FOR BODY SCRUBS

(Available at your local health food store)
- Natural bristle dry brush
- Almond Oil
- Olive Oil
- Sea Salt
- All food ingredients listed can be purchased in a grocery store.

- **HEALING TUB TREATS**
Indulge in these healing bath recipes whenever you have 30 minutes to relax.

1. Apple cider vinegar can help relieve dry, itchy skin. Pour one cup apple cider vinegar into a tub of warm water. Soak for 20 minutes. Do not rinse skin. Simply towel off.

2. Milk is a wonderful exfoliator for all skin types including those with eczema or dry skin. Lactic acid in milk exfoliates and evens the skin tone. Fat in milk moisturizes the skin. Pour two gallons

of whole milk in a tub of hot water. Cold milk cools the bath water considerably so be sure to fill the tub with hot water. If you have oily skin, use non-fat milk. You may also substitute milk with two cups of powdered milk in a tepid tub of water. Relax in the bath for 20 minutes. Rinse with tepid water.

3. For a soothing bath or for those with eczema, steep 4 to 5 chamomile tea bags in 3 cups boiling water. Remove tea bags, and add tea to tepid tub water. Tannins in chamomile can help relieve inflammation or itching, dry skin. Don't rinse, just towel off.

4. Morton Salts™are non-toxic salts that can help draw out excess fluids and relax aching muscles and feet. Add 6 – 12 cups of Morton Salts™to tepid tub water.

5. To make a luxurious bath oil combine 1 tbsp. almond, olive or grape seed oil, 2 drops lavender essential oil and 3 capsules Vitamin E. Massage into skin, then sit in a tub of warm water. Rinse off.

6. To condition and moisturize dry or mature skin, combine 3 tbsp. jojoba oil with 6 drops frankincense essential oil. Massage into skin and sit in a tub of warm water. Frankincense softens, heals and prevents wrinkles, stimulates cell regeneration, is an anti-inflammatory and moisturizer.

7. For stiff muscles or sore back, add 12 drops thyme and 5 drops eucalyptus essential oil to bath water.

8. Add one bottle of hydrogen peroxide and 2 lbs. Morton

Salts™ to warm tub water. Soak for 20 minutes. This recipe is used by models and actresses to shed toxins and water weight quickly. Morton Salts™ draw out excess fluids.

BEST BEAUTY BUYS TUB TREATS

(Available at your local health food store)
• Apple Cider Vinegar
• Essential Oils
• Powdered Milk
• Grape Seed Oil
• Jojoba Oil
• Frankincense Oil
• Vitamin E capsules
• Morton Salts (grocery store)

• **BODY MOISTURIZERS**
Skin is the body's largest organ which is why I prefer to moisturize with natural oils. *NOTE:* Natural oils can go rancid quickly so make body oil recipes in small batches and place unused oils in the refrigerator to keep fresh until needed. After bathing or showering, apply oil on clean skin to seal in moisture. Below are some effective body moisturizers you can make.

1. I use this one every day. It's one of my favorites. Combine ½ bottle of almond or grape seed oil and 1 tsp. of fragrant essential oil. I like china lilly, rain or musk. You can find essential oils at health food stores and "body" or scent shops.

2. For mature or dry skin add 2 to 3 drops frankincense essential oil to recipe #1. Frankincense is an anti-inflammatory

125

and cell regenerative that is beneficial to those with mature or dry skin. You can also combine Egyptian frankincense oil with distilled water and spray on the body

3. Shea butter, coconut and avocado oil are also excellent body moisturizers, however almond and grape seed oil absorb more quickly which means you can get dressed immediately.

4. Jojoba oil is also suggested for dry skin or dry scalp, however this one takes a while to absorb so it would not be my first choice.

BEST BEAUTY BUYS BODY MOISTURIZERS

(Available at your local health food store)
- Frankincense Essential Oil
- Vitamin E Capsules
- Almond Oil
- Grape Seed Oil
- Shea Butter
- Coconut Oil
- Jojoba Oil

- **PREVENTING CELLULITE**

Cellulite occurs when collagen fibers under the skin and around fat cells become trapped with fluids and toxins. As we age collagen weakens, fat and toxins herniate through the damaged collagen and dimpled skin occurs. Exfoliating skin regularly can help stimulate collagen and help drain the lymphatic system. If you have cellulite, or want to prevent it, consider the following:

Leg & Body Care

1. You've heard this a million times — Drink 8 to 10 glasses of water daily. Cellulite and water retention are signs that you're not drinking enough water. You will not lose body fat, toxins or diminish cellulite unless you drink sufficient water daily. Drinking at least 64 oz. of water a day can help eliminate water retention and body fat. (see Slimming Secrets for water and fat-reducing facts). Water retention causes bloating, constipation, irritability and exacerbates cellulite. If you don't like water, add some fresh lemon juice for a more refreshing taste. Or try chamomile, cat's claw, or green tea to increase circulation as well as help reduce inflammation and bloating.

2. Eating a 'good' fat and low-carbohydrate diet can help burn body fat and prevent fluid retention.

3. Daily dry brushing can help exfoliate skin, boosts circulation of the blood, drains the lymphatic system and releases toxins. Dry-brush cellulite-prone areas using a natural bristle brush before showering. Dry-brush toward the heart using a C-shaped motion. Locate cellulite-prone areas in front of the mirror then dry brush those areas for 30 seconds. Start at wrists working up to shoulders. Then start at ankles and brush up legs. Brush buttocks and tummy. When done correctly your skin should be slightly pink. Do not brush areas with cuts, rashes or sunburn. Shower with tepid water.

4. Skin rolling is a somewhat unheard of massage that has actually been around for over 20 years. This unusual rolling and pinching of the skin can help break up cellulite and fat deposits, stimulates the skin and helps detoxify and sculpt the body. You'll be amazed at how much dead skin comes off your body during skin rolling. Exfoliating skin helps stimulate collagen production which helps keep the body looking more firm and youthful too.

5. Two or more times weekly, massage cellulite-prone areas (thighs, tummy and buttocks) using an electric massager or even a rolling pin, to help break down cellulite. Or try chopping strokes (hands in a karate-like position), moving up and down the fatty areas of the thighs and buttocks. Kneading the skin is also beneficial.

6. The elastic in regular underpants cuts off lymphatic circulation and congests fluids, fat and toxins, causing cellulite. To prevent lymphatic congestion and cellulite, try switching to wearing thong underwear no underwear at all.

7. Calcium/Magnesium supplements, Vitamin E and Evening Primrose Oil can aid in weight loss and also help ease bloating and water retention. Check with your doctor before taking supplements.

8. Endermology® is a non-surgical treatment that uses suction and rolling motion as it glides over skin to help rupture fat cells. It works at the blood level of the skin, draining the lymphatic system, mobilizing the skin and massages the various levels of tissue down to the muscle. Endermologie® can help break up scar tissue under the skin, which can improve results after liposuction or plastic surgery. It's FDA approved for reducing cellulite and requires about 20 sessions to achieve results. A monthly session is required to maintain results. Sessions cost from $75 to $125 each. It's even more effective when combined with ultrasonic treatments (see #9).

9. For more stubborn cases of cellulite or if you want to achieve smoother-looking thighs, consider an "ultrasonic" treatment in conjunction with Endermologie® (vacuum massage). This

combination is one of the most effective non-invasive methods of reducing and smoothing dimpled-looking skin. NOTE: Ultrasonic treatment is a type of ultrasound, however it differs from that used in ultrasound imaging or physiotherapy. Ultrasonic treatment's warm heat waves penetrate into the subcutaneous (fat) layer only. It helps smooth the skin by softening or breaking up the fatty deposits, promotes lymphatic drainage and releases hardened connective tissue. The treatment is followed with Endermologie®. Look for salons that offer Dermosonic® treatments. This is becoming a popular treatment for cellulite reduction in spas.

10. VelaSmooth by elos™ is a recent revolutionary technology that combines Infrared Light and Bi-Polar Radio Frequency to help smooth dimpled areas. Radio frequency heats the adipose tissue and infrared light heats the subcutaneous fat and helps stimulate elasticity of the skin. This treatment involves a vacuum or suction which helps smooth out the skin and helps drain the lymphatic system. Results are reported to be superior.

11. Mix 2 cups sea salt with ½ cup almond or olive oil. After showering stand in the shower and apply salt scrub to wet thighs and buttocks. Rub in a circular motion using your hand or a nylon exfoliating body glove. Rinse with tepid water.

12. Bentonite clay draws out impurities and tightens skin. In a glass bowl combine equal parts water or apple cider vinegar with bentonite clay. Stir to a paste consistency and apply to cellulite-prone areas. Let dry. You will feel a tightening or pulling sensation. Wash clay off in the shower with tepid water.

13. While standing on newspaper, apply warm caffeinated coffee grinds onto thighs, tummy and buttocks. Most of the

grinds will fall to the ground, leaving a caffeine-rich, moist, brown residue. Caffeine is the active ingredient that reduces the appearance of cellulite. Wrap moistened areas with cellophane. After 30 minutes, remove cellophane and brush any excess grinds onto the newspaper. Shower off thighs and buttocks while scrubbing the areas using a face cloth, baking soda or loofa. This remedy is a little messy - but it's a quick fix way to help temporarily diminish cellulite.

14. For quick, temporary relief of unsightly cellulite apply Cellulite Eraser. Within minutes it can help flatten out the dimpled look of cellulite and lasts for several hours. Go get your bikini!

15. Cellulite creams that contain retinol, glycolic or salicylic acid can help smooth and firm skin by stimulating collagen and elastin production. Relastyl(TM) Deep and Fine Line Wrinkle Repair can be applied to thighs as well.

16. Self-tanner can help camouflage cellulite. Some of the most famous lingerie models use self-tanner for this reason. Yes even models have to battle or conceal cellulite.

17. Mesotherapy is known to help diminish cellulite. It involves injecting a series of natural and pharmaceutical medicines into the cellulite-prone areas. This treatment has been around for decades in Europe and South America and is fairly new to the United States. I've seen some cases that showed some good results, however there's no hiding this treatment from your spouse or partner as severe bruising can last for weeks and a minimum of six or more treatments are required. Best results are seen when combined with ultrasonic. Prices range from $350 to $500 an area/per session.

BEST BEAUTY BUYS FOR PREVENTING CELLULITE

(Available at your local drug store)
- Dry Brush
- Morton Salts
- Retinol Treatments for Cellulite
- Calcium, Magnesium, Evening Primrose, Vitamin E
- Self-Tanner

(Available at your local health food store)
- Dry Brush
- Sea Salts
- Morton Salts (at your grocery store)
- Cat's claw, green & chamomile tea
- Bentonite Clay
- Essential Oils

(To order visit www.hollywoodbeautysecrets.com)
- Cellulite Eraser™

Resources:
- Los Angeles, Endermologie® combined with Ultrasonic, 310-821-3354
- Brentwood, CA. Fountain of Youth Med Spa, Dermosonic™ 310-914-8772
- Go to Dermosonic™ on the www to find a spa/practitioner
- Los Angeles, CA. VelaSmooth, Comprehensive Cosmetic, 310-268-2288
- Go to www.syneron.com to find a VelaSmooth by elos™ spa/practitioner.
- Marina del Rey, CA. Skin Rolling and training contact C. Weatherman, 310-823-6796

131

Part Seven

- West Los Angeles, CA. Skin Rolling. Contact Jackie Lee 310-390-4719

Mesotherapy:
- Newport Beach, CA. Dr. S. Jennings, 949-717-4811
- Fountain Valley, CA. Dr. E. Llorente, 714-885-8980

• AFFORDABLE WAYS TO RELIEVE SPIDER VEINS

1. Combine one part witch hazel and one part horse chestnut oil. Rub mixture into spider vein areas.

2. Combine one part horsetail herb and two parts witch hazel. Rub mixture into spider vein areas.

3. Rub Vitamin K cream or Arnica cream into spider vein areas. Try AOK crème by Age Advantage.

4. Powerful, topical Perfect RX Perfect LEGS contains haloxyl and Vitamin K to effectively help fade spider veins.

5. Standing all day causes blood to pool in the legs, creating spider or varicose veins. To prevent spider veins, put feet up at the end of the day.

6. Uncross your legs!

7. Sclerotherapy can also help diminish spider and varicose veins, however there is some down time. See an experienced Phlebologist. Also check out Telangitron® and Irodex Diode Laser Treatments for spider veins in "Anti-Aging Alternatives".

BEST BEAUTY BUYS FOR SPIDER VEINS

(Available at your local drug store)
- Witch Hazel
- Horse Chestnut oil
- Horsetail Herb

(To order visit www.hollywoodbeautysecrets.com)
- A-O-K Crème by Age Advantage
- Perfect RX Perfect Legs

- **FADING SCARS**
1. Scars are the body's natural response to burns, scrapes, surgery, acne and more. Scar Gel can be used on newly healed wounds or old scars to make them look softer, smoother and less noticeable. The active ingredients help break down scar tissue and encourage cell renewal. This process of breakdown and renewal helps diminish the discoloration associated with scars. The result is that scars are softened, flattened and their appearance is markedly diminished as they blend in with surrounding tissue. Scar Gel works on old, new, keloid, acne, burn or surgery scars. If a scar is lumpy or bumpy or has discoloration, this product will be of benefit. You can also use Scar Gel on stretch marks to help fade the reddish or purplish color that many stretch marks exhibit. Scar Gel is superior to Vitamin E oil, is non-oily and non-greasy so it won't stain your clothes. It contains allantoin to help heal and soften the skin and aid in tissue building, panthenol to increase skin suppleness and onion extract (allicin), an anti-bacterial, anti-fungal and anti-viral. Apply twice daily, or more for two to six months to see

maximum results. This product is a top seller.

2. Acne and Scar Crème by Age Advantage can also help fade acne scars, wounds and burns. This revolutionary formulation penetrates into the second skin layer, addressing scar tissue damage from the inside out. It contains glycolic acid to help exfoliate the surface scar tissue.

BEST BEAUTY BUYS FOR SCARS

(To order visit www.hollywoodbeautysecrets.com)
- Scar Gel by Derma e
- Acne & Scar Crème by Age Advantage

• DIMINISHING STRETCH MARKS
Over 80 million Americans are confronted with stretch marks. The following products can help flatten or help fade the blue, red or purplish color that many stretch marks exhibit.

1. Scar Gel is a top selling natural formulation containing extracts that can help fade blue, red and purplish stretch marks. Scar Gel is superior to Vitamin E oil and is non-oily and non-greasy so it won't stain your clothes. Scar Gel contains allantoin to help heal and soften the skin and aid in tissue building as well as panthenol to increase skin suppleness. (Read more about Scar Gel above.)

2. Another product called Stretch Mark Crème™ is a healing crème that can be safely worn during pregnancy. It contains oils, antioxidants, collagen, elastin, vitamins and glycolic acid to help smooth and diminish the appearance of stretch marks.

3. Combining shea or cocoa butter with lemongrass essential oils can help tighten skin and help fade blue or purple-color stretch marks. NOTE: DO NOT APPLY essential oils if pregnant. This recipe is for use AFTER pregnancy ONLY.

4. A topical stretch mark cream called StriVectin-SD™ has been clinically proven to reduce the depth, length, texture and uneven pigmentation associated with stretch marks. It stimulates collagen production which thickens and firms skin. Apply it three times a day for four to six weeks to see results. StriVectin-SD™can also be used on the face and around the eyes to diminish fine lines and wrinkles.

BEST BEAUTY BUYS FOR STRETCH MARKS

(To order visit www.hollywoodbeautysecrets.com)
- Scar Gel Creme by derma e
- StriVectin-SD™
- Stretch Mark Crème™ by Age Advantage

Boost Your Metabolism

ANTI-AGING SUN CHLORELLA

(Check with your physician before taking supplements listed)

Incredible anti-aging and nutrient-packed supplement Sun Chlorella is a super toxin-fighter and immune-booster that can help turn back the clock and energize your body. Within weeks you'll have more energy and you'll see lines, wrinkles and age spots diminishing, pores tightening, smoother skin, improvement with dry skin or adult acne and you'll have a rosier, healthier complexion. It also improves and strengthens nails and can help hair become more shiny and soft. This is one of my Hollywood beauty secrets as well as that of many celebrities and doctors.

Sun Chlorella is a single-cell freshwater green algae that is a rich source of nucleic acid. It helps your body reproduce immune cells to help you feel energized and can help keep you youthful-looking. Sun Chlorella can help alleviate digestion or stomach problems, can help stop weight gain, diminishes joint pain and can help banish pigmentation spots. Sun Chlorella can help your body renew itself by fighting off premature aging and contains 18 amino acids that protect your body's defenses. It includes cystine, T-cell building arginine and Lysine. Sun Chlorella can also:

- aid in weight loss and help clear skin. When fat cells become clogged with toxins, the system becomes sluggish, constipated, blemished and weight gain is inevitable.

- help cleanse cells of fatigue-causing toxins that rob you of energy. You will have more energy and your mood will be uplifted.
- help increase oxygen to the cells. Many experience relief of asthma, fatigue, joint pain, stiffness and swelling.
- help keep you regular and prevent bad breath. It contains the highest amount of chlorophyll of any plant.
- can help protect your system from hormonal imbalances.
- help maintain healthy cholesterol levels, better circulation and blood pressure

For more information and **a free sample of Sun Chlorella, call 1-800-595-6776.** Tell them Hollywood Beauty Secrets referred you.

TRIPHALA
(Check with your physician before taking any supplements)

The Hindus say, "If you don't have a mother, Triphala will take care of you." This fruit-derived herb can be taken regularly for overall health. It is considered one of the greatest internal herbal cleansing formulas. Even children and those with irritable bowel syndrome have been known to benefit from Triphala. However, check with your doctor first.

Triphala is known to help:

- regulate and unclog the stagnating liver and intestines
- improve digestion and circulation
- lower cholesterol and blood pressure
- cleanse the blood and liver

- prevent sickness
- relieve constipation
- relieve eye diseases such as cataracts or glaucoma
- control chronic weight gain.
- is a systematic rejuvenative, colonic tonic and cleanser
- contains 30% linoleic acid (omega-6 fatty acids)
- contains tannins (anti-inflammatory agents) which can help
prevent bladder infections and relieve arthritis
- contains anti-viral properties, which can help prevent colds

(Available at your local health food store)
- Triphala by Solaray

• REMEDY BLOATING

The following supplements can help relieve bloating. Check with your physician before taking the suggested supplements.

1. Drinking eight to 10 glasses of water a day helps prevent bloating. I increased my water intake for three days, lost three pounds and my tummy flattened.

2. Supplements such as 1000 mg. Calcium/Magnesium, evening primrose oil (omega -6 fatty acid) Vitamin E and borage oil can help prevent bloating and can assist in weight loss.

3. Total EFA (essential fatty acids) is a supplement containing flax seed, borage seed and fish oil. It moisturizes skin and eases bloating. Flax ignites fat burning and can slow down the aging process.

4. Teas such as chamomile, mint, ginkgo biloba, green and cat's claw can help remedy bloating and stimulate circulation. Green tea helps metabolize fat.

5. Chewing gum can cause gas and bloating.

6. Avoid bread and starches as they cause water retention and bloating. Avoid salt and diet sodas that contain sodium. If you must have soda try Hansen's Diet Soda. It has zero sodium.

7. Combining papaya and garlic tablets before each meal creates a diuretic effect.

8. Constipation causes bloating and weight gain. Drink at least 8 to 10 glasses of water daily. Water flushes toxins and fat and promotes regularity. See more benefits of water in "Significant Slimming Secrets" in this section.

9. Increasing fiber intake can help prevent constipation and bloating. Triphala, an herbal fruit blend, regulates a sluggish liver and intestines. Triphala is taken with meals. Read more about Triphala a few pages back.

10. Sun Chlorella can also help boost your metabolism, helps protect your immune system and much more. Read more about Sun Chlorella at the beginning of this chapter. Eating fiber-rich cereal, fruits and veggies, fiber capsules or flax oil supplements can help promote regularity and prevent bloating. Be certain to drink at least eight to 10 glasses of water daily to push fiber through the system. Otherwise fiber may cause a blockage and bloating.

11. Dandellion tea can help prevent fluid retention, detoxifies the liver, prevents gallstones, and can clear blemishes as it is a blood purifier.

12. Dairy contains lactose. Many adults have lactose intolerance, which causes bloating. If you can't part with dairy, try a lactase enzyme to prevent bloating. Or substitute cow's milk with soy, almond or rice milk. These "milk substitutes" are calcium-fortified.

13. Enzyme deficiencies can cause bloating and indigestion. Consider taking digestive enzymes such as bromelain, pineapple, papain, papaya or lactase. Beano® is another good one. Each enzyme mentioned above can break down either fat, fiber, protein or milk sugar (lactose) which aids digestion. Enzymes can also eliminate gas, bloating and other digestive problems. Consider taking a broad spectrum blend of enzymes before meals so all foods are broken down with just one pill. Broad spectrum enzymes break down fat, fiber, protein, carbohydrates and milk sugar. See a physician or homeopathic doctor for proper doses.

BEST BEAUTY BUYS TO REMEDY BLOATING

(Available at your local health food store)
- Flax Seeds
- Total EFA by Health From the Sun (essential fatty acids),
- Triphala by Solaray
- Citrucel Fiber Caplets
- Beano®
- Lactase Enzymes

- Essential Enzymes by Source Naturals (broad spectrum digestive enzymes)
- Sun Chlorella – for a free sample call 1-800-595-6776
- Go to www.lifescript.com for customized supplements.

● **RELIEVING CONSTIPATION &
SLUGGISH METABOLISM**
Frequent constipation can cause weight gain, gas, bloating and discomfort. If you have pain, see your physician. The following suggestions may be helpful:

1. Flax seeds and flax seed oil can help regulate the bowels. Before bed mix two to three heaping tbsp. ground flax seeds with 3/4 glass of water. Stir and drink. Follow with a full glass of water. If you don't like the taste of flax seeds, take flax seed oil capsules.

2. Citrucel® (methylcellulose) is another effective, soluble fiber that does not cause bloating, cramps or gas often associated with other types of fiber. Take Citrucel caplets as directed on the bottle to regulate your system.

3. Drinking one glass of carbonated water daily can help reduce constipation. Also include drinking a minimum of 10 glasses of regular water daily to promote regularity.

4. Salmon, evening primrose oil, and fish oils contain omega-6 and omega-3 fatty acids which can help ease bloating and keep the system lubricated and healthy.

5. High-protein diets lack fiber. Eat vegetables, nuts and low glycemic fruits such as blueberries, strawberries and raspberries

for fiber. Have at least one leafy green salad each day as well as two to four servings of green beans, asparagus, broccoli, artichokes or brussel sprouts. And drink plenty of water to push fiber through the body (minimum 10 glasses daily).

6. Read about Triphala and Sun Chlorella mentioned at the beginning of this chapter. Both can assist in relieving constipation and a sluggish metabolism.

7. For immediate relief of constipation, insert a glycerin suppository. If you have pain or discomfort, skip #7 and see your doctor immediately. *NOTE:* If you are taking fiber caplets and eating fiber-rich foods and are still bloated or constipated you must increase your water intake in order to push the fiber through your system.

BEST BEAUTY BUYS FOR CONSTIPATION & SLUGGISH METABOLISM

(Available at your local health food store)
- Flax seeds
- Flax oil supplements
- Triphala by Solaray
- Sun Chlorella

(Available at your local drug store)
- Glycerine Suppositories
- Benefiber®
- Citrucel ® Caplets

• SIGNIFICANT SLIMMING SECRETS
(Check with your physician before trying these slimming secrets.)

1. Reduce fat with water! We've heard it a million times — drink eight glasses of water a day. Once you read these amazing fat loss facts, I guarantee you'll increase your water intake! After I did the research, I increased my water intake for three days and guess what? — I lost three pounds and my tummy stayed flat all day long. I no longer experienced bloating. Drinking sufficient water has been proven to be one of the easiest and most affordable ways to lose body fat. Here's why:

- Water helps the body naturally metabolize fat and eliminate toxins.
- Your kidneys need water to function properly. When the kidneys don't have enough water, the liver has to take over some of the work of the kidneys and you'll likely gain weight.
- It's the liver's job to metabolize fat, but if it has to do the additional work of the kidneys, the liver can't do its job sufficiently. The result? The body slows fat metabolization and you stop losing weight!!
- Drink 64 oz, that's eight - 8 oz. glasses of water a day. When weather is hot, when exercising, or if you're overweight, you will need to drink additional water. For every 25 pounds of additional weight you are carrying, consume another 8 oz. glass of water. (i.e. If you're 40 to 50 pounds overweight, you need to add two more glasses of water to your daily intake. If you're 75 pounds overweight, add three glasses, and so on. Check with your physician.

143

- Water helps keep your muscles and skin looking toned and tight. Water helps hydrate the muscles. When you lose weight, particularly larger amounts, your skin will sag. However, if you increase your water intake while losing weight, water can help prevent saggy looking skin. When skin cells are hydrated with water, your skin looks more tight and firm.
- Water helps suppress your appetite. Drink a glass of water when you feel hungry between meals. Cold water is even better. It supposedly enters the system more quickly and can help burn more calories.
- Water binds to salt. If you consume a lot of salt, to stop water retention you must drink even more water.
- Water helps eliminate toxins and most importantly, fat! While dieting, the fat you're metabolizing needs to leave your body. Increasing water flushes out the fats, toxins and waste.
- You won't lose weight if you're constipated. Stop constipation by drinking more water. When you increase your water intake, you'll regulate bowel movements which can help decrease body fat.

2. You can help fight fat and may even help protect your health with apple cider vinegar and Kyolic garlic. Many individuals have been known to lose inches, pounds and prevent infections or sickness with this simple slimming beverage. My parents are living proof that this recipe can work. They lost about 15 to 20 lb. each and both have kept the weight off for four years now. May I add that my parents used to suffer from stomach problems, indigestion and ulcers and since taking this beverage, they no longer suffer from stomach or indigestion problems. Of course, always check with your doctor before taking new remedies, supplements or trying diet tips, especially if you are on any type of medication or have any health problems. Don't do

this if you're pregnant or breast feeding unless you check with your doctor. Apple cider (AC) vinegar contains 19 minerals including potassium, phosphorus, magnesium, calcium, sulfur and iron. Apple cider vinegar can help jump-start the metabolism and it's loaded with amazing health benefits.

Apple cider vinegar can:
- help kick the metabolism into fat-burning mode,
- help regulate water balance and prevent fluid retention,
- promote healthy cell and tissue growth,
- protect against potent bacteria and viruses such as colds and flus,
- help diminish a sore throat,
- help thin and lower blood pressure,
- promote oxygenation of the blood,
- help destroy fungi and protect you from food poisoning,

When you combine apple cider vinegar with Kyolic (odorless) garlic, this powerful tonic flushes fats out of your system, helps your body fight infections and even some cancers. Russian doctors administer garlic to their colon and stomach cancer patients. You can take regular garlic capsules as well.

Benefits of garlic:
- can help lower cholesterol and blood pressure,
- can help keep weight down,
- eliminates yeast overgrowth,
- can help prevent heart attacks and strokes by preventing a build-up of plaque and fatty deposits in the arteries,
- helps prevent certain diseases. It has over 200 disease-fighting compounds relating to Herpes I, Herpes II, parasites, bacteria, and fungu,
- is an antiseptic and has antibiotic effects,
- can help reduce blood fat and blood sugar,
- can help promote wound healing,
- has no side effects,

- safe to use on a long-term basis.
- can help eliminate blemishes.

Apple Cider Vinegar and Kyolic Garlic Recipe

NOTE: Check with your doctor before taking this beverage. Add 1 tbsp. apple cider vinegar to 8 or 10 oz. or water. You can use either organic or regular apple cider vinegar. Take two (approx. 100 to 200 mg.) Kyolic odorless garlic capsules or tablets with the vinegar/water drink. Drink this combination before each meal (breakfast, lunch and dinner). If the vinegar mixture is too strong, start with 1 tsp. of apple cider vinegar. If you still can't tolerate the taste, try adding one tsp. of raw honey to the water and vinegar and warm slightly in the microwave and drink it down with the Kyolic garlic capsules. If you're not fond of drinking the AC vinegar, have two salads a day using AC vinegar and olive oil dressing. And simply drink the Kyolic garlic capsules three times a day with a glass of water.

3. Fact: Did you know that diets low in fat (less than 10%) can increase your likelihood of having a stroke by 50%? The tiny arteries of the brain need a sufficient amount of 'good' fat to keep arteries strong, thus prevents ruptures or bleeding. When reading food labels look for 'good' fats such as unsaturated, monosaturated or polyunsaturated. 'Good' fats include oils such as virgin or cold-pressed olive, canola, grape seed, flaxseed and sunflower oil. Nuts such as almonds, walnuts, hazelnuts and brazil nuts are 'good' fat choices. Eating unsaturated fats can help reduce risk of colon, lung, breast and prostate cancer, cardiovascular disease and can help you lose weight too! Avoid saturated, hydrogenated or transfatty acids such as margarine, fast or fried foods, red meat, butter, lard or shortening and palm oil. These fats can increase cholesterol and risk increase of colon and breast cancer.

4. Keep a food diary. Jot down everything that you eat, including snacks and you'll soon identify any bad eating habits.

5. Eat a diet rich in complex carbohydrates (vegetables, whole grains and low glycemic fruits, fish and poultry. Vegetables and fruits also help curb your appetite as they are fiber-rich, thus filling. Dark-colored fruits and vegetables contain more antioxidants and can help reduce the risk of many diseases and cancers. Excellent low-glycemic fruit choices include blueberries, strawberries, blackberries, raspberries, red grapes, apples, nectarines, peaches, plums, cantaloupe and tomatoes. Excellent vegetable choices include: broccoli, red or green cabbage, green beans, asparagus, swiss chard, leafy lettuce, kale, spinach, and sweet potatoes. Beans and legumes are high in fiber and also contain protein. Fish is a wonderful protein choice as it has about 50% less calories than red meat and 30% less calories than poultry. Fish is also high in omega-three fatty acids and protein. Try to consume fish two to three times a week. Cook fish in olive oil and lemon for maximum nutrition. Avoid high-glycemic carbohydrates such as sugar, white flour breads, pasta, rice, beets, potatoes, syrups, corn sweeteners, cakes, cookies, candy, rice cakes, popcorn, chips, crackers, juice, soda and alcohol. These foods raise insulin levels in the blood stream which stimulates fat cells to store more fat. Foods that trigger high insulin levels may also contribute to high blood pressure, heart attack, stroke and adult diabetes.

6. Never miss a meal. When you skip breakfast or lunch, the liver produces more LDL in the blood and that raises bad cholesterol. You'll also be more likely to overeat at your next meal or have too many snacks. Did you know that snackers or

'grazers' often take in more calories than if they'd had three square meals a day?

7. Eat less at night. Did you know that you burn about 15% less calories at night than in the day? Your metabolism slows down and overeating or snacking will cause stored fat. Make lunch the largest meal of your day. This way you will burn it off by the time dinner roles around.

8. Drink 10 glasses of water a day. Carbonated water can also aid in weight loss.

9. Hypothyroidism (underactive thyroid) can make losing weight difficult. Have your thyroid checked by your doctor.

10. Stress releases corticosteroid hormones (cortisol) which prevents weight loss and can add extra inches around the abdomen. Regular exercise blocks cortisol production. Talk to your doctor about a supplement called Relora™ which can block cortisol production. Rescue Remedy™oral spray can also ease stress.

11. Calcium can aid in weight reduction and help prevent osteoporosis. Recommended dose is generally 1000mg daily. Try OsteoMax calcium supplements which do not cause gas like many others.

12. Flax seeds and flax oil supplements can help ignite fat burning and balance hormones. Take flax seed supplements with meals or grind flax seeds and sprinkle over salad or cereal.

13. For years European women have been taking green tea

extract supplements for fat metabolism. Green tea extract is a natural thermogenic (fat burner) and antioxidant. And green tea can help stimulate collagen production which firms skin.

14. Carbohydrate blockers can neutralize over 60% of the starch eaten in a meal. Combined with a sensible diet and regular exercise, you may lose up to two pounds a week. Effective starch blockers contain a kidney bean extract known as phaseolus vulgaris or Phase 2 Starch Neutralizer. The bean extract prevents starch from breaking down into sugar in the system. Starch leaves the body through the intestines.

15. Bladderwrack (another name for seaweed or kelp), fish and shellfish, are high in iodine. The thyroid captures iodine from the blood stream, which speeds the metabolism and can aid in weight loss. ParKelp (TM), a bladder wrack seasoning, may be added to your favorite meats, chicken, fish or veggies. Have your thyroid checked before taking bladderwrack.

16. To lose weight you must walk at least 35 to 45 minutes a day to speed up your metabolism. Take a 35-minute walk during your lunch hour with a co-worker, then walk an hour each day on the weekend. Walking while talking burns more calories. Walking up steps is easier than lunges, provides great aerobic exercise and firm, sexy legs. Walk or ride your bike to do your errands. On the weekend, walk to breakfast, the library or your local coffee shop.

17. Lifting weights increases muscle mass and stimulates the body's own growth hormone production which can help keep skin looking toned, firm and more youthful-looking. The more muscle you have, the more calories you'll burn. It's imperative to add weight lifting or weight resistance exercises to your workout

regimen, especially at age 40 or over, as growth hormone production dramatically declines, causing more body fat and loss of elasticity in skin. Resistance exercises can help prevent sagging skin. If you're uncomfortable going to a conventional gym, check out one of the Curves® Circuit-training facilities across America. The regimen involves a series of weight resistant exercises that are completed in 30 minutes. Brilliant concept and a comfortable non-threatening workout environment. Suitable for women of all ages.

18. Pilates is also another great anti-aging alternative and one of the best exercises for quick results. This regimen of controlled movements, which are done on either a mat or a reformer, is ideal for targeting, tightening and toning problem areas in just weeks. Developed by Joseph Pilates, many dancers, athletes, models, celebrities and even physical therapists use Pilates to quickly heal, strengthen and tone the body. Pilates classes are very popular and very affordable. See the best deal in town below.

19. Order my "Under 30-Minute Model Sculpting Workout" for weight resistence exercises that you can do in the privacy of your own home. All you need is a chair and a set of 3 lb. weights. This is the personal workout that has kept my figure in model shape for the past 20-plus years. Do this challenging workout three to five times a week and you'll see and feel a difference in your body in just four weeks. The Bar Method is another exercise video I highly recommend. It is a series of dance, yoga, and isometric exercises that quickly sculpt the body.

20. Lack of sleep and exercise can decrease the body's natural production of human growth hormone. When growth hormone

declines, abdominal fat and reduced muscle mass are inevitable. If you have trouble sleeping or are not able to get to the gym as often as you'd like, consider Symbiotropin™. It's a synergistic blend of amino acids that ensures a sound sleep, lean muscle mass, weight loss, revitalized hair, firm skin, wrinkle prevention, and stronger nails. You'll awake rested and feel an increase in energy during the day. Millions upon millions of people take Symbiotropin™. Many individuals report looking and feeling younger and having more energy in just eight weeks.

BEST BEAUTY BUYS FOR SLIMMING

(To order visit www.hollywoodbeautysecrets.com)
- Sympbiotropin™
- OsteoMax ™Calcium
- Thermo Green Tea Extract
- Under 30-Minute Model Sculpting Workout
- Bar Method Video

(Available at your local health food store)
- Flax Seeds
- ParKelp™ Seasoning
- Relora™
- Rescue Remedy™ by Bach (oral spray)
- Starch Away (Carbohydrate Blocker)
- Go to www.lifescript.com for custom formulated supplements.

Resources:
- Los Angeles, CA. Best Deal in Town!! Pilates Classes & Privates, Beyond Physical Therapy, 310-578-5960

PMS & Balancing Hormones Naturally

- **RELIEVING PREMENSTRUAL SYNDROME (PMS)**

Taking the following supplements 10 days before your menstrual cycle may help relieve bloating, weight gain, moodiness and cramps associated with PMS. Check with your doctor before taking supplements or changing your diet.

1. Calcium (1000 mg. daily) can help prevent mood swings and irritability, soothes low back pain and cramps, reduces food cravings, aids in weight loss, bloating, excess water weight gain and prevents osteoporosis. OsteoMax™ is a superior calcium supplement that can help prevent osteoporosis. For those who cannot swallow supplements easily, OsteoMax™is a convenient effervescent drink that can help fight diseases that age bones, joints and loss of collagen. It helps increase bone density and is absorbed into the body more efficiently than regular calcium supplements.

2. Magnesium (360 mg. 3 times daily) can battle bloating, ensures a sound sleep and reduces night time leg cramps.

3. Flax seed oil supplements can help balance hormones.

4. Vitamin E can ease bloating, headaches, depression and tender breasts.

5. Evening primrose oil and black current oil can help ease bloating, swelling and cramps.

6. Exercise triggers the endorphins (neurotransmitters in the

brain) which raises serotonin levels. Increased serotonin levels act as natural "feel good" mood boosters in the brain. Take a daily walk if you can't get to the gym.

7. ProEndorphin is a fantastic natural mood booster that's loaded with essential B vitamins (anti-stress), amino acids, DMAE and herbs that provide increased energy. It's ma huang-free. Taking ProEndorphin 10 days before menstruation or as a mid-day pick-me-up, helps trigger a positive mood and energy within 15 minutes. Oz Garcia, a top celebrity trainer, gives ProEndorphin to his clients to provide energy and endurance before a workout.

8. Sam-e (S-Adenosylmethionine), an amino acid, is a highly effective mood booster that can help with sadness, anger, moodiness or depression. Sam-e has many other benefits and no known side effects. It supports joint health, brain function, healthy connective tissue, cleanses the liver and can help slow the aging process by protecting DNA. DO NOT use Sam-e if you suffer from manic depression (bi-polar) or are currently taking anti-depressants. Ask your doctor about Sam-e. For full potency make certain Sam-e is enteric coated and in a blister pack (not a bottle). Take on an empty stomach. **Check with your doctor before taking Sam-e.**

9. Topical natural progesterone creams are known to help promote hormone balance within the body. Apply progesterone cream or serum to the abdomen, inner arms or thighs. Use as directed on label for PMS. **Do not use progesterone cream if you are taking hormone replacement therapy (HRT's).**

BEST BEAUTY BUYS FOR PMS

Supplements:
(To order visit www.hollywoodbeautysecrets.com)
- OsteoMax™ Calcium
- ProEndorphin™

(Available at your local health food store)
- Vitamin E, Primrose & Black Current Oil supplements
- Flax Seed supplements
- Sam-e by Jarrow

Progesterone creams:
(Available at your local health food store)
- Nugest 900™ and Nugest Serum™
- Visit www.lifescript.com for custom formulated supplements.

- **HELPFUL PERIMENOPAUSAL TIPS**
Around age 35 women start experiencing signs of perimenopause that include hormone imbalances, bloating, weight gain, moodiness, sadness or depression. Popular books on perimenopause include "Could It Be Perimenopause?" by L.S. Asher Goldstein, "Before The Change: Taking Charge of Your Perimenopause," by Ann Louise Gittleman, "Screaming To Be Heard: Hormone Connections Women Suspect and Doctors Ignore," by Elizabeth Lee Vliet, M.D. Suzanne Summers book, "The Sexy Years", is a must-read. It's loaded with great information about bio-identical hormones. Check with your doctor about these natural alternatives supplements, as some can effect blood pressure:

1. Consider taking a daily multiple vitamin containing folic acid. Try Vitrin, a multivitamin that contains 29 essential vitamins and minerals, the antioxidant equivalent of five servings of fruits and vegetables.

2. Consider taking 500 milligrams of Vitamin C or Vitamin Ester-C twice daily.

3. Consider taking a daily Vitamin B complex which has 50 milligrams of B6. Vitamin B5 can help support and revive the adrenal glands which produce and secrete estrogen, adrenaline, DHEA, testosterone, cortisol, and pregnenoline. Take Vitamin B5 with breakfast or lunch to give you energy later in the day. Ask your doctor about doseage. NOTE: B5 must be taken with a multi-vitamin, otherwise it can deplete the body of other vitamins.

4. Consider taking 400 I.U. of Vitamin E daily.

5. Flax oil supplements and seeds can help balance hormones, ignite fat burning, slow the aging process, keep skin hydrated and youthful-looking and help promote regularity. Take flax supplements twice daily.

6. Consider taking 1000 milligrams of Calcium/Magnesium daily. OsteoMax™, a calcium supplement, is highly recommend for preventing osteoporosis. For those who cannot tolerate swallowing supplements, OsteoMax™ effervescent tablets dissolve quickly in water and do not cause gas like other calcium supplements.

7. Calcium D-Glucarate can help balance excess estrogen. It's of particular benefit to women suffering from hormone imbalances, those who have a history of breast cancer or are using birth control pills. Consuming foods rich in Calcium D-Glucarate can help. They include apples, broccoli, grapefruit and cherries.

8. Soy-rich foods such as soy beans, tofu, soy cheese, soy powder, soy nuts and soy milk are rich in phytoestrogens that help balance estrogen in the system.

9. Visit www.drhirani.com to learn more about balancing hormones naturally.

10. Applying topical, natural progesterone cream can help alleviate hormone imbalances. Read more on progesterone cream in "What Your Doctor May Not Tell You About Menopause: Balance Your Hormones and Your Life from Thirty to Fifty," by John R. Lee, M.D., et al. And "The Sexy Years" by Suzanne Sommers.

11. ProEndorphin™ is a fantastic, natural mood booster that's loaded with essential B vitamins, amino acids, DMAE and herbs to provide increased energy. When I feel stressed I take ProEndorphin™. Within 15 minutes I feel terrific. Celebrities and supermodels take ProEndorphin™ for instant energy or before working out. It is stimulant-free.

12. Sam-e (S-Adenosylmethionine), an amino acid, is a highly effective mood booster that can help with sadness, anger or depression during this stage of your life. It has been used in Europe for over 20 years to treat mild depression. To read more

about the benefits of Sam-e see "Relieving Premenstrual
Syndrome (PMS)" #8.

*BEST BEAUTY BUYS FOR BALANCING
PERIMENOPAUSAL HORMONES*

Supplements:

(To order visit www.hollywoodbeautysecrets.com)
• Vitrin Multivitamin
• OsteoMax™ Calcium Supplements
• ProEndorphin™

(Available at your local health food store)
• Flax Seeds and Flax Oil supplements
• Calcium D-Glucarate by Tyler
• Sam-e by Jarrow

Progesterone Creams:
(Available at your local health food store)
• Nugest 900™ and Nugest Serum™

• RELIEVING HOT FLASHES & MENOPAUSE
Going through menopause is a special time in a woman's life. As
our body chemistry changes, shifts in hormones occur. Women
often don't know what to expect but knowing the signs can help
us and our loved ones to understand what we will be going
through. With menopause, no two women are alike. We all
develop various levels of testosterone, estrogen and
progesterone in our systems at different times each month. So
taking dong quai, chaste tree, wild yam root and soy may not
necessarily help you. These common menopausal supplements

may have helped your best friend but your hormone levels will differ from hers. The best way to help yourself get through menopause is to read everything you can so you can make educated decisions. Here are some popular books on menopause: "What Your Doctor May Not Tell You About Menopause," by John R. Lee, M.D. and "The Wisdom of Menopause", by Christiane Northrop, M.D. I also highly recommend Suzanne Sommers' book, "The Sexy Years." It's a wealth of knowledge if you have questions about bio-identical hormones. She really knows her stuff and offers resources (doctors and compounding pharmacies) in the book. You can also learn more about balancing hormones naturally at www.drhirani.com.

Always check with your doctor before taking any supplement.

Here are some suggestions that are known to help:

1. A daily multivitamin, up to 2000 milligrams of buffered Vitamin C daily, up to 800 IU of Vitamin E daily, 500 milligrams of Magnesium at night or a calcium/magnesium supplement.

2. Osteoporosis is a major concern for women, especially as we age. OsteoMax™has a unique calcium delivery system that prevents bone disease, joint problems and loss of collagen. This calcium supplement that does not cause gas, like some calcium supplements.

3. Soy, lentil, lima and kidney beans contain phytoestrogens called isoflavones which act like the body's natural estrogen to stabilize and help suppress hot flashes. Eat one to two servings of phytoestrogen-rich foods daily including; soy beans, roasted soy nuts, soy cheese, soy yogurt, soy milk (have a soy latte),

tofu stir-fry. Avoid alcohol and spicy foods. Sun Chlorella (see "Boost Your Metabolism") can also help balance hormones.

4. Calcium D-Glucarate can help balance excess estrogen. It's particularly beneficial to women suffering from hormone imbalances or those who have a history of breast cancer. Foods rich in Calcium D-Glucarate are apples, broccoli, citrus fruits and cherries.

5. Taking flax seeds or flax oil supplements can help balance hormones, slow down aging, ignite fat burning and help keep skin youthful and supple. While conducting interviews with several women, I discovered many who experienced few uncomfortable signs of menopause. Their diets consisted of flax seeds, essential fatty acids (EFA's), colorful vegetables and fruits, soy products, nuts, fish and greatly reduced meat and chicken consumption. In addition they advised women to keep busy, not be too self-absorbed and live each day focusing on other areas of our lives as menopause is a perfectly natural stage. Great advice - something to think about!

6. Stop smoking and avoid caffeine in the afternoon or evening.

7. Exercise regularly. Try walking, deep breathing and yoga.

8. Chinese medicine and acupuncture is a natural, drug-free treatment. It can be of great help with balancing hormones and other signs associated with menopause such as loss of libido, backache, fatigue, graying hair, hair loss and vaginal dryness.

9. Applying natural progesterone cream daily, when not taking hormone replacement therapy (HRT's), has helped many individuals reduce hot flashes and vaginal dryness. Read more

on progesterone cream in "What Your Doctor May Not Tell You About Menopause," by John R. Lee, M.D.

10. Ask your doctor about Sam-e (S-Adenosylmethionine), a natural mood booster. To read more about the benefits of Sam-e see "Relieving Premenstrual Syndrome (PMS)".

11. For energy and mood uplifting, as well as energy and weight loss, consider taking Sun Chlorella. For more on Sun Chlorella see "Boost Your Metabolism".

12. The Journal of American Medical Association reports that some antidepressants (selective serotonin reuptake inhibitors) such as Paxil™ and Prozac™ can boost serotonin levels. Women experienced 50% relief of hot flashes, mood swings and sadness decreased, and they experienced more energy when taking Paxil. These products may have some side effects so I would take them as a last resort. Talk to your physician.

BEST BEAUTY BUYS FOR RELIEVING HOT FLASHES & MENOPAUSE

Supplements:
(To order visit www.hollywoodbeautysecrets.com)
- Vitrin™ Multivitamin
- OsteoMax™ Calcium Supplements
- Flax Seeds and Flax Oil Supplements

Other Products Recommended:
(Available at your local health food store)
- Pro-Gest™ Body Cream by Emerita
- Sam-e by Jarrow

Hair Care

• HEALTHY HAIR TIPS FOR ALL HAIR TYPES

1. For healthy, lustrous hair consume foods rich in protein and healthy oils including essential fatty acids, fish, olive and grape seed oil, and nuts. Include a variety of colorful vegetables, fruits and whole grains in your diet. Sun Chlorella, an algae from Japan, is known to help add more shine and soften hair. For a free sample of Sun Chlorella call 1-800-595-6776 or find it at your local health food store.

2. Choose shampoos that moisturize, are gentle, or contain UV protectants, formulated for your hair type (normal, oily, dry). Always use conditioner on ends of hair. Use cool water when rinsing hair. This closes hair follicles and adds shine. A top selling shampoo/conditioning product that's popular amongst hollywood celebrities is WEN Fig Cleansing Conditioner. Developed by Chaz Dean, a top colorist in Hollywood, this all-in-one cleansing and conditioning shampoo does not contain sodium laurel sulfates which are found in almost all shampoos. Sodium laurel sulfates can fade and strip color, cause dull, dry, brittle hair, can damage the scalp and may even cause hair loss. Chaz developed WEN without the use of detergents or harsh chemicals. And the beauty of this product is that it can be used by EVERY hair type!! Whether you have delicate ethnic hair, fine, coarse, medium, dry, oily, color-treated or chemically damaged hair, this product is for you. It helps color last longer, adds sheen, moisture, luster, strength and manageability to even chemically-treated hair. In addition, it helps stimulate the scalp promoting circulation which can help stop hair loss and promote

healthier hair growth. See the Best Beauty Buy list to order WEN Fig Cleansing Conditioner.

3. Do not scrunch hair or rub hair with a towel after washing as this creates tangles and makes combing more difficult. Instead, very gently squeeze out excess water and wrap hair in a towel.

4. Use a wide-toothed comb or fingers to gently comb through hair.

5. Before blow drying, apply a silicone-infused product to protect hair.

6. Use a medium heat setting to blow dry hair. Hold dryer four inches away from hair to prevent damage. Finish drying with a blast of cool air to close hair follicles and add shine. Consider investing in an ion blow dryer. The ions in the warm air break down water molecules and lock in moisture. Ion dryers dry hair faster, preventing dry, frizzy or damaged hair.

BEST BEAUTY BUYS FOR HEALTHY HAIR

(Products are available at your local beauty supply or drug store unless otherwise noted)

Shampoo/Conditioner:
(To order visit www.hollywoodbeautysecrets.com)
• WEN Fig Cleansing Conditioner

More Shampoo Choices:

• Paul Mitchell® Super Skinny Daily Shampoo
• Redkin® All Soft Shampoo

- Pantene® Pro-V Shampoo with UV filters
- L'Oreal® Color Vive Shampoo with UV filters

Serums:
- L'Oreal® Vive Smooth-Intense Anti-Frizz Serum with silicon
- Biosilk® Silk Therapy
- Frizz Ease by John Frieda

Other Products Recommended:
- Vidal Sassoon Ionic Hair Dryer
- Conair Ion Shine Hair Dryer

• STOP FLY AWAY HAIR
One of the best remedies for fly away hair is Aveda™ Elixir Leave-In Conditioner. After shampooing, towel-dry hair and add elixir. Comb through hair. Leave in and then blow dry.

BEST BEAUTY BUYS FOR FLY AWAY HAIR
(Available at your local beauty supply store)
- Aveda™ Elixir Leave-In Conditioner

• DIMINISHING DANDRUFF OR DRY SCALP
Try one of these remedies for a dry scalp:
1. Place two peppermint tea bags and ½ cup apple cider vinegar in a bowl. Add one cup boiling water. Let cool and place in a plastic bottle. Use as a final rinse after shampooing.

2. Mix 1 cup witch hazel with 4 drops rosemary essential oil. After shampooing hair, rub liquid onto scalp.

3. Shampooing with hot water can cause a dry scalp or dandruff. Use tepid water.

4. Separate hair using a comb. Apply olive oil between sections on scalp. Wait 30 minutes then shampoo as normal. Follow with the rinse in #1.

5. Shampoo containing 2% salicylic acid or zinc can calm eczema or dry scalp.

6. Add peppermint essential oil to regular shampoo.

7. Apply a liquid scalp treatment containing 3% salicylic acid to remedy dandruff, seborrheic dermatitis or psoriasis.

8. Consider investing in an ion blow dryer. The ions in the warm air break down water molecules, locking in moisture while preventing dry scalp or frizzy hair. Because they dry hair faster, ion dryers create less damage than conventional dryers.

BEST BEAUTY BUYS FOR DRY SCALP

(Available at your local health food store)
- Peppermint Tea
- Apple Cider Vinegar
- Rosemary Essential Oil
- Peppermint Essential Oil
- Witch Hazel
- Olive Oil

Shampoos:
(Available at your local drug store)
- Selsun® with 2% salicylic acid
- Neutrogena® T/Gel Overnight Dandruff Treatment with salicylic acid
- Head and Shoulders® (zinc-based shampoo)
- Nizoral® (zinc-based shampoo)
- Vidal Sassoon Ionic Hair Dryer
- Conair Ion Shine Hair Dryer

Other Products Recommended:
(To order visit www.hollywoodbeautysecrets.com)
- WEN Fig Cleansing Conditioner

- **REPAIRING DRY OR COLORED HAIR**
1. Choose moisturizing shampoos that do not contain sodium laurel sulfates (which are found in almost all shampoos). Sodium laurel sulfates can fade and strip color, cause dull, dry, brittle hair, can damage the scalp and may even cause hair loss. A top hollywood hair stylist developed WEN Fig Cleansing Conditioner without the use of detergents or harsh chemicals. And the beauty of this product is that is can be used on EVERY hair type!!! Whether you have ethnic hair, fine, coarse, medium, dry, color-treated or chemically damaged hair, this product is for you. It helps color last longer, adds sheen, moisture, luster, strength, manageability and hydrates hair. In addition, it helps stimulate the scalp promoting circulation, can help stop hair loss and promotes healthy hair growth.

2. Shampoo hair with tepid (warm) water and finish with a cool rinse to close hair follicles and add shine.

3. Use conditioner before shampooing for hydration and manageability. Apply conditioner to dry hair first, and work into hair with a little water. Wait 5 to 10 minutes then shampoo hair.

4. Apply a silicone-infused product prior to blow drying to protect hair. Hold dryer four inches away when drying. After drying, blast hair with cool air to close follicles and add shine to hair.

5. Consider investing in an ion blow dryer. The ions in the warm air break down water molecules, locking in moisture. This prevents dry, frizzy hair, heat damage and dry scalp.

6. Two times a week apply an intensifying conditioner such as olive oil or hot oil treatment to ends of hair. Wear a shower cap. Leave on for 15 minutes then shampoo as normal. Use cold water as a final rinse to close follicles and add shine.

7. Massage 1 to 2 tbsp. mayonnaise onto scalp down to ends of hair. The oil in mayonnaise conditions hair, vinegar maintains pH of hair and closes hair follicles, creating shine. Wear a shower cap for 10 to 30 minutes. Then shampoo as normal. For added shine use cold water as a final rinse.

8. Before swimming or spending time in the sun, comb UV protectant conditioner through hair to keep it hydrated and protected.

BEST BEAUTY BUYS FOR DRY OR COLORED HAIR

(Products are available at your local beauty supply or drug store unless otherwise noted)

Shampoos:
(To order visit www.hollywoodbeautysecrets.com)
- WEN Fig Cleansing Conditioner

- Paul Mitchell® Instant Moisture Daily Shampoo
- BedHead® Moisture Maniac Shampoo
- Joico® Reconstructor Shampoo

Deep Conditioners:
- Infusium 23 Leave-In Treatment
- Redken® Extreme Heavy Cream Deep Fuel Conditioner
- Alberto VO5® Hot Oil Hair Treatment
- St. Ives™ Hot Oil Treatment

(To order visit www.hollywoodbeautysecrets.com)
- WEN Fig Cleansing Conditioner

Other Products Recommended:
- L'Oreal® Vive Smooth-Intense Anti-Frizz Serum with silicone
- Banana Boat Hair & Scalp Spray with SPF 15
- Pantene® Pro-V Repair and Protect Restoration Treatment

- **PREVENTING SPLIT ENDS**
1. For split ends a trim is suggested.

2. Choose moisturizing shampoo with UV filters.

3. To protect hair from split ends use a leave-in, heat activated conditioner or serum.

4. For a temporary quick fix, mix half a mashed ripe avocado with 4 drops lavender essential oil. Shampoo hair then massage mixture from middle to ends of hair. Leave on for 20 minutes. Rinse with cool water to close follicles and create shine.

5. Blow dry hair using an ion hair dryer. The ions in the warm air break down water molecules, locking in moisture, preventing dryness and causing less damage.

BEST BEAUTY BUYS FOR SPLIT ENDS

(Products are available at your local beauty supply or drug store unless otherwise noted)
Shampoos:
* Rusk® Calm Shampoo
* BedHead® Control Freak Shampoo

(To order visit www.hollywoodbeautysecrets.com)
* WEN Fig Cleansing Conditioner

Serums:
* Biosilk® Silk Therapy

Conditioners:
* Redkin® All Soft Conditioner
* Joico® K Pac Reconstructor Condtioner
* Rusk® Calm Conditioner

(To order visit www.hollywoodbeautysecrets.com)
- WEN Fig Cleansing Conditioner

Other Products Recommended:
- Vidal Sassoon Ionic Hair Dryer
- Conair Ion Shine Hair Dryer
- Lavender Essential Oil

- **VOLUMIZING THIN, LIMP, LIFELESS HAIR**

1. Choose a volumizing shampoo and apply light weight conditioner on ends of hair only.

2. To add bounce and body to hair, allow one cup of beer to become flat at room temperature. After shampooing rinse hair as normal. Then massage beer through hair. Leave in for two to three minutes. Rinse with cool water.

3. Apply a volumizer or a root-lifting product to roots before blow drying.

4. When blow drying, hang head upside down. Dry hair on medium heat. When finished, use a blast of cold air to seal follicles and add shine.

BEST BEAUTY BUYS FOR THIN, LIMP, LIFELESS HAIR

(Products are available at your local beauty supply or drug store unless otherwise noted)

Volumizing Shampoos:
- Sebastian® Mohair Volumizing Shampoo
- Matrix™Amplify Volumizing System
- Catwalk™ Thickening Shampoo
- Dove® Volumizing Shampoo with Weightless Moisturizers

Other Products Recommended:
- Matrix Amplifying Volumizing System Conditioner
- Thermasilk® Maximum Control Mousse
- TRESemme® Hydrology Boosting Moisture Mousse
- Aussie® Real Volume Root Lifter Volumizing Styler
- Clairo®l Herbal Essences Natural Volume Root Volumizer

- **STRAIGHTENING CURLY HAIR**
1. After shampooing, apply a silicone-infused product or serum to prevent frizzy hair.

2. While hair is wet, pull it back into a tight pony tail to straighten roots. Leave hair in a pony tail as long as possible or until hair is dry.

3. When blow-drying, use a large-barreled round brush to hold hair taut. Invest in an ion blow dryer to prevent frizzies and dryness.

4. After blow drying go over any wavy areas using a ceramic straightening iron. Ironing seals hair follicles and creates shiny hair.

5. Finish with a moisture barrier to prevent moisture from entering hair follicles.

BEST BEAUTY BUYS FOR STRAIGHTENING CURLY HAIR
(Products are available at your local beauty supply or drug store unless otherwise noted)

Frizz Erasers:
- L'Oreal® Vive Smooth-Intense Anti-Frizz Serum with Silicone
- Biosilk® Silk Therpay
- Paul Mitchell® Straight Works
- Redken® Outshine Anti-Frizz Polishing Milk
- Therasilk® Shine and Shape Gel
- Physique® Keep It Straight Lotion
- Frizz Ease Moisture Barrier by John Frieda

Conditioners:
- Redken® Extreme Heavy Cream Deep Fuel Conditioner
- Joico K Pac Reconstructor Condtioner
- Neutrogena® 60 Second Intensive Conditioner
- Sebastian® 911 Deep Conditioner

Other Products Recommended:
- Vidal Sassoon Ionic Hair Dryer
- Conair Ion Shine Hair Dryer
- Visit a beauty supply shop for a professional, ceramic straightening iron.

• CARING FOR CURLY OR ETHNIC HAIR
1. Choose hydrating shampoos that do not contain sodium laurel sulfates which can fade and strip color, cause frizzy, dry, and brittle hair. A hollywood colorist and stylist developed WEN Fig

Cleansing Conditioner without the use of detergents or harsh chemicals. And the beauty of this product is that is can be used by EVERY hair type!! Whether you have ethnic hair, fine, coarse, medium, curly, straight, dry, color-treated or chemically damaged hair, this product is for you. It helps color last longer, adds sheen, moisture, luster, strength and manageability to the hair. In addition, it helps stimulate the scalp promoting circulation, can help stop hair loss and promotes healthy hair growth.

2. To banish frizz, scrunch curl defining gel or hair serum into damp hair. Allow hair to air dry and separate with fingers.

3. Texturizing glaze is a leave-in style cream that does not flake. Apply it to damp hair.

4. Use a diffuser on medium or low when blow drying hair. Consider investing in an ion hair dryer to lock in moisture and prevent dry, frizzy hair.

BEST BEAUTY BUYS FOR CURLY HAIR
(Products are available at your local beauty supply or drug store unless otherwise noted)

Shampoos & Conditioners:
- KMS® Curl Up Shampoo and Conditioner
- L'Oreal® CurlVIVE Curl-Moisture Shampoo

(To order visit www.hollywoodbeautysecrets.com)
- WEN Fig Cleansing Conditioner

Serums:
- John Freida Frizz-Ease Dream Curls
- Biosilk ®Silk Therapy
- L'Oreal® Vive Smooth-Intense Anti-Frizz Serum with Silicone

Gel:
- Sebastian® Wet
- Let's Jam Shining & Conditioning Gel
- L'Oreal® Studio Line Curl Defining Gel

Other Products Recommended:
- Alterna Texturizing Glaze
- Vidal Sassoon Ionic Hair Dryer
- Conair Ion Shine Hair Dryer

• REMOVING BUILD-UP FROM HAIR

1. Combine 1 tsp. baking soda with 1 tbsp. regular shampoo. Use this mix to shampoo hair. For added shine, use cold water as a final rinse. After drying, blast hair with cool air. This closes follicles and creates shine.

2. Use a clarifying shampoo that does not strip or dry hair.

Part Ten

BEST BEAUTY BUYS FOR REMOVING
BUILD-UP FROM HAIR

Build-up Eliminators:
**(Products are available at your local beauty supply or drug
store unless otherwise noted)**

- Baking Soda
- KMS® Daily Fixx Clarifying Shampoo
- Terax Latte
- Pantene® Pro-V Purity Clarifying Shampoo

- **TIPS FOR SHINY HAIR**
1. For shiny hair, choose WEN Fig Cleansing Conditioner. This
two-in-one shampoo/conditioner does not contain sodium laurel
sulfates which can fade and strip color, cause dull, dry, brittle
hair, damage the scalp and may even cause hair loss. WEN Fig
Cleansing Conditioner adds sheen, moisture, luster, strength and
manageability to the hair. In addition, it helps stimulate the scalp
promoting circulation, can help stop hair loss and promotes
healthy hair growth. Chaz Dean developed WEN Fig Cleansing
Conditioner without the use of detergents or harsh chemicals.
And the beauty of this product is that is can be used by EVERY
hair type!! Whether you have ethnic hair, fine, coarse, medium,
dry, color-treated or chemically damaged hair, this product will
help add shine and luster to your hair. Dozens of celebrities use
this fantastic product. See the Best Beauty Buy list for WEN Fig
Cleansing Conditioner.

2. Combine ½ cup apple cider vinegar with 2 cups water in a
plastic bottle. After shampooing, rinse hair as normal,
then do a final rinse using the vinegar/water mixture.

Follow with an extra cool rinse for super, shiny hair.

3. Apply shine infuser, serum or silicone-based products to hair for shine. Use serum that is formulated for your hair type.

4. After blow-drying, finish with a blast of cool air to seal follicles and add shine.

BEST BEAUTY BUYS FOR SHINY HAIR
(Products are available at your local beauty supply or drug store unless otherwise noted)

(To order visit www.hollywoodebautysecrets.com)
- WEN Fig Cleansing Conditioner

Shampoos:
- TreSemme® Vitamin-C Deep Cleansing Shampoo
- Alterna® Hemp Shine Shampoo
- Sebastian® Laminates Shampoo

Conditioners:
- Alterna Hemp Shine Conditioner
- Sebastian® Laminates Conditioner

(To order visit www.hollywoodebautysecrets.com)
- WEN Fig Cleansing Conditioner

Other Products Recommended:
- Apple Cider Vinegar
- Therasilk® Shine and Shape Gel
- Concair Headcase Frizz Serum Lusterizer
- Neutrogena® Instant Shine Detangler

- L'Oreal® Vive Smooth Intense Anti-Frizz Serum with Silicone

- **TOP HAIR SPRAY CHOICES**

A favorite hair spray choice of many Beverly Hills hair stylists is Aerogel by Triprofessional Haircare. It has the flexibility of a gel and holds the hair in place without a stiff or sticky feeling. Here are more of the favorites used by the pros:

BEST BEAUTY BUYS FOR HAIR SPRAY

(Products are available at your local beauty supply or drug store unless otherwise noted)

Light Hold:
- Paul Mitchell® Super Clean Light
- Sebastian® Zero G
- Linea Shapee

Medium Hold:
- Goldwell® Trend Line
- Sebastian® Shaper

Strong Hold:
- Aerogel(TM) by Triprofessional Haircare
- Pantene® Pro-V Volumizing Hairspray Maximum Hold (all-day volume for hard-to-hold hair)
- Redken® Inflate Volumizing Finishing Spray
- Sebastian® Shaper Plus

- **ELIMINATING BRASSY HAIR**

1. To help diminish brassy hair or highlights, pour cream or whole milk onto hair. Leave on for 10 minutes. Lactic acid in milk can help neutralize the color.

2. Choose hydrating and UV protectant shampoos and conditioners that prevent fading color.

3. Apply UV protectant conditioner or UV spray on hair before spending time outdoors. Rinse hair after swimming in the ocean or pool.

4. WEN Fig Cleansing Conditioner is a non-foaming shampoo and conditioner in one that can help prevent brassy hair. It also adds shine, hydrates, and helps hold color in the hair.

BEST BEAUTY BUYS FOR BRASSY HAIR

(Products are available at your local beauty supply or drug store unless otherwise noted)

Brass Eliminators:

- Aveda™ Blue Malva
- Artec™ White Violet Shampoo
- Biolage® Color Care Shampoo
- Clairol® Shimmer Light

(To order visit www.hollywoodbeautysecrets.com)
- WEN Fig Cleansing Conditioner

UV Protectant Products:
- Pantene® Pro-V Color Care Shampoo, Conditioner, Mousse and Spray with UV filters
- Artec® UV Conditioner
- L'Oreal® Color Vive Shampoo and Conditioner with UV filters
- Banana Boat Hair & Scalp Spray with SPF 15

• PREVENTING FADED HAIR COLOR

1. Sun causes oxidation, which fades hair color. Using shampoos that contain sodium laurel sulfates can strip hair and fade color. WEN Fig Cleansing Conditioner is free of sodium laurel sulfates. It's a top seller that does not strip color from hair and it can help add sheen, luster, strengthen and hydrate colored hair.

2. Use color-enhancing shampoo to refresh color and choose hair coloring products that are fade-resistant.

3. Apply UV protectant conditioner or spray before spending time outdoors or swimming.

BEST BEAUTY BUYS FOR FADED HAIR COLOR

(Products are available at your local beauty supply or drug store unless otherwise noted)

Shampoos & Conditioners:
- Biolage® Color Care Conditoner

- Artec® Color Depositing Shampoo
- Artec® UV Conditioner
- Neutrogena® Clean Color Defending Shampoo and

Conditioner
(To order visit www.hollywoodbeautysecrets.com)
- WEN Fig Cleansing Conditioner

Fade Resistant Hair Color and UV Protectants:
- Clairol®Natural Instincts Hair Color
- L'Oreal® Superior Preference Fade Resistence Color UV-Protectant
- Banana Boat Hair and Scalp Spray with SPF 15

• DIMINISH THINNING AND RECEDING HAIR

1. For thinning or receding hair, remarkable WEL Vitalizing Shampoo and Scalp Stimulator are creating quite a buzz in California. Developed by a doctor of internal medicine, this shampoo can help slow or reduce hair loss in three to four weeks and can help grow voluminous hair in just three to four months.

This chemical-free formulation contains vitamins, herbs, trace minerals and marine extracts. Whether hormonal, disease-related thinning or receding hair, this formulation can help provide new volume and hair length. Using Vitalizing Shampoo on its own is highly effective, however, for thinning or receding hair, use both shampoo and stimulator. Both products can be used by women AND men. Use daily or every other day.

2. Silica gel is known to help speed hair growth as well as help grow thicker hair and strengthen nails. Many books have been written about the powers of silica gel. Combining prenatal

vitamins, silica gel and WEL Vitalizing Shampoo has helped many achieve more rapid hair growth. Check with your physician on brands of prenatal vitamins. Maturna™ was a brand that one model swore by when she combined it with silica gel.

BEST BEAUTY BUYS FOR THINNING/RECEDING HAIR

(To order visit www.hollywoodbeautysecrets.com)
- WEL Vitalizing Shampoo & Scalp Stimulator

(Available at your local health food store)
- Silica gel
- Prenatal vitamins

• VOLUMIZING HAIR WITH CLIP-ON EXTENSIONS
Name a female celebrity that's frequently seen on the red carpet, and you can be almost certain she's sporting clip-on hair extensions. Everyone in Hollywood seems to be clipping volumizing natural hairpieces into their hair. If you want this look, be sure to buy human hair extensions as they are easier to manage and comb through.

BEST BEAUTY BUYS FOR CLIP-ON HAIR EXTENSIONS

(Available at your local beauty supply shop)
His & Her Hair on Wilshire, Los Angeles

Medicine Cabinet

• **PREVENTING & EASING HEARTBURN**

Reflux from the stomach into the esophagus occurs when there is a dysfunctional lower esophageal sphincter. As food sits undigested in the stomach, the acid from the stomach comes up the esophagus, causing heartburn. The following remedies are known to help relieve heartburn, however check with your doctor before trying them:

1. Did you know that the reason many of us get heartburn is because we don't have enough acid to help digest food? This remedy has helped my parents both lose weight and help prevent heartburn and may I add, that they no longer suffer from ulcers or stomach ails. Add 1 tbsp. apple cider vinegar to an eight to 10 oz. glass of water and drink before each meal. The acid in the vinegar helps digest food. NOTE: If you already heartburn, DO NOT do this.

2. Drink a glass of water 15 minutes before a meal.

3. Suck on a lozenge or chew gum before and after a meal to stimulate saliva whichs helps rinse the esophagus.

4. Besides being unhealthy, smoking causes heartburn.

5. Chew food slowly and thoroughly.

6. Eat several small meals a day. Eating large meals, particularly your last meal of the day, can cause heartburn.

7. Digestive enzymes, taken before meals, can assist digestion. Choose broad-spectrum enzymes which have enzymes that break down fats, carbs, protein, fiber and milk sugar.

8. Avoid peppermint, wine, caffeine and fatty foods. Limit chocolate and sweets. Chocolate in particular can exacerbate heartburn.

9. Stop eating at least two to three hours before bedtime. Lying down causes undigested food to come up the esophagus.

10. Limit alcohol to two drinks a day.

11. Some prescriptions can cause heartburn. Check with your pharmacist or doctor.

BEST BEAUTY BUYS FOR EASING HEARTBURN

(Available at your local health food store)

- Essential Enzymes™by Source Naturals (broad spectrum digestive enzymes)
- Apple Cider Vinegar

- **EASING ACID REFLUX**
1. To buffer acid in the esophagus, stimulate saliva production by chewing gum or sucking on a piece of candy before or after a meal. Saliva rinses the esophagus.

2. See the remedies listed on the previous pages which can help relieve heartburn.

3. If natural alternatives don't work, ask your doctor about prescription Protonix®, Prevacid® or Nexium®.

• **RELIEVING MIGRAINE HEADACHES**
Migraines are prompted when blood vessels constrict, causing a reduction in oxygen, nutrients and blood supply to the brain. Many elements can trigger a migraine including stress, tension, hormonal changes that occur during menstruation, post-pregnancy, peri-menopause and menopause. Decreased levels of magnesium and riboflavin can trigger a migraine. Foods such as nitrate-rich products (salami, hot dogs, sausage, bacon, pork), artificial sweeteners, caffeine, wine, alcohol, aged cheeses and chocolate can also trigger migraines. Talk to your doctor before attempting any of the following remedies:

1. Aerobic exercise oxygenates the bloodstream and stimulates the endorphins. If you can't get to the gym, take a daily 20-minute walk during your lunch break.

2. A daily intake of 300 mg. of magnesium can help dilate blood vessels and stimulates seratonin (feel good neurotransmitters). Magnesium is often combined with calcium supplements, which are typically taken by women on a daily basis.

3. A daily intake of riboflavin (Vitamin B2) can ease the pain, occurrence and/or duration of migraines. Foods rich in B2 include: fortified cereals, breads and milk.

4. A daily intake of CoQ10, is known to help reduce the number of monthly migraine attacks considerably.

5. A daily intake of 100 mg. Feverfew™ a natural anti-inflammatory, can help reduce pain, nausea and duration of a migraine.

6. Ginger ale calms nausea, a symptom of migraines. Ginger is available in capsule form or try drinking ginger ale or tea.

7. Avoid trigger foods noted above.

8. Botox®** injections can prevent certain types of migraines. Contact a neurosurgeon for more information. (**Botox® is a registered trademark of Allergan, Inc.)

BEST BEAUTY BUYS FOR RELIEVING MIGRAINES

(Available at your local health food store)
• Supplements listed above.
• Go to www.lifescript.com to order custom supplements.

• **RELIEVING ARTHRITIS**
1. It's common for women to experience arthritis in their hands as they age as this may be due to frequently exposing hands to water (doing dishes, laundry and housework). Be sure to wear rubber gloves whenever working with water to help prevent arthritis.

2. To help reduce fluid build-up, and relieve joint pain try a product called JointTastic™ It's a highly concentrated topical creme that transports key ingredients such as Glucosamine, MSM, Chondroitin, Arnica Montana, Aloe Gel and Emu Oil.

JointTastic is medically proven to work. It reduces inflammation and pain associated with arthritis. Worn nightly, many individuals report benefits within three weeks use.

3. Triphala, a fruit derivative, and the enzyme Bromelain, derived from pineapple, are natural anti-inflammatories that can help revelieve arthritis.

4. Cayenne (capsicum annum) found in Ben Gay (TM) creates circulation to provide arthritic relief.

5. L.E.D. Light Therapy can help reduce the pain of arthritis. A home light therapy unit is now available. Contact louisa@hollywoodbeautysecrets.com for more information.

BEST BEAUTY BUYS FOR RELIEVING ARTHRITIS

(To order visit www.hollywoodbeautysecrets.com)
- JointTastic™ Topical Crème

- **PREVENTING A YEAST INFECTION**

If you suspect a yeast infection, see your doctor. You will likely be prescribed a vaginal suppository or oral treatment. The following remedies may help prevent a yeast infection. Check with your doctor before taking these supplements.

1. Avoid insulin-inducing foods including starches such as sugar, potatoes, pasta, bread, cereal, rice, and beets, peas, corn, all sweets and high-glycemic fruits.

2. Stick to a diet rich in low-glycemic fruits including strawberries, blueberries, raspberries, watermelon, kiwis and cantaloupe. Fill up on fiber, vegetables and leafy greens to keep your system regular and flush out yeast.

3. Eat yogurt regularly or take acidophilus supplements in the morning on an empty stomach The bacterial cultures can help reduce your risk of yeast infections.

4. Garlic can help fight yeast overgrowth. Consider taking Kyolic (odorless) garlic as it is less offensive than regular garlic.

5. If you have a yeast infection, taking garlic supplements containing 4000 mcg. active allicin up to three times daily may help. See your doctor.

6. Caprylic acid supplements and grapefruit seed extract can also attack yeast. Place two drops grapefruit seed extract in a gelatin capsule and drink with a glass of water two times a day. Take caprylic acid capsules as directed on the bottle.

7. As a preventative measure, taking olive leaf extract starting five days before your menstrual cycle is known to help prevent yeast. Olive leaf extract is an anti-fungal.

BEST BEAUTY BUYS FOR YEAST PREVENTION

(Available at your local health food store)
- Caprylic Acid
- Liquid Concentrate Grapefruit Seed Extract
- Gelatin Capsules

- Optimal Nutrients® Garlic 4000
- Olive Leaf by Solaray
- Go to www.lifescript.com for custom formulated supplements.

• PREVENTING BLADDER & URINARY TRACT INFECTIONS

1. If you suspect a bladder or urinary tract infection, see your doctor immediately.

2. Eating blueberries, cranberries and cherries can help prevent bladder and urinary tract infections. These fruits are loaded with tannins that attack infection-causing bacteria. Drinking cranberry or black cherry juice can help flush out the infection. Dilute these juices with water if watching caloric intake or buy unsweetened juices.

3. Triphala, an herbal fruit supplement, contains 45% tannins as well as anti-inflammatory and anti-viral properties. Triphala can be taken with daily meals.

4. Olive Leaf Extract, an anti-viral, anti-bacterial and antifungal, may help reduce bladder and urinary tract infections.

4. Uva Ursi is known to help reduce urinary tract infections.

BEST BEAUTY BUYS FOR BLADDER INFECTIONS

(Available at your local health food store)
- Triphala by Solaray
- Uva Ursi by Nature's Way

- Olive Leaf by Solaray

- **FADING SCARS**

1. Acne and Scar Crème™ penetrates deep into the dermal layer of the skin to stimulate new skin cell growth. It also exfoliates the top layer of skin as it contains salicylic acid. This is a top seller that is known to help fade acne scars, burn scars, wounds and surgical scars. If scar is exposed to sun, top with sunscreen daily to prevent darkening.

2. To help fade dark scars try products containing hydroquinone (bleaching cream) and wear sunscreen over the area as skin will be sensitive to the sun.

3. Retin-A can help speed cell regeneration which helps diminish scars over time. Apply creams containing Retin A or Vitamin A or simply try rubbing papaya on scars regularly. Papaya is nature's natural Retin-A. Apply sun screen overtop of scars daily.

4. Scar Gel is not a concealer but a scar treatment. This is a top selling product. Scars are the body's natural response to burns, scrapes, surgery, acne and more. Scar Gel can be used on newly healed wounds or old scars to make them look softer, smoother and less noticeable. The active ingredients help break down scar tissue and also stimulate cell renewal which helps diminish the discoloration associated with scars. With consistent use scars will blend in with surrounding tissue. Scar Gel works on old, new, keloid, acne, burn or surgery scars. If a scar is lumpy or bumpy or has discoloration, this product will be of benefit. You can also use Scar Gel on stretch marks to help

remove the reddish or purplish color that many stretch marks exhibit. Scar Gel is superior to Vitamin E oil, is non-oily and non-greasy so it will not stain your clothes. Scar Gel contains: allantoin to help heal and soften the skin and aid in tissue building; panthenol to increase skin suppleness; onion extract (allicin) an anti-bacterial, anti-fungal and anti-viral. It takes anywhere from two to six months of twice-a-day applications to see maximum results.

5. Use concealer to camouflage scars. Dermablend® Body Cover can dramatically conceal scars.

6. Plain or soy yogurt can help fade pigmentation spots. Apply either to scars for 10 - 15 minutes four times a week.

7. Lasers can reduce some types of scar pigmentation. See a laser center or get a referral from your dermatologist.

8. Mineral makeup can nicely camoflauge some scars.

BEST BEAUTY BUYS FOR FADING SCARS

Exfoliating Cream:
(To order visit www.hollywoodbeautysecrets.com)
- Acne and Scar Crème by Age Advantage
- Scar Gel by derma e
- Alpha Lipoderm with Green Tea Extract by Derma e

Bleaching Products:
(Available at your local drug store)
- Palmers™ Skin Success Fade Cream with 2% hydroquinon
- Esoterica® Fade Cream also contains hydroquinone

Other products recommended:
- Plain or Soy Yogurt
- Sheercover™ Mineral Makeup. To order call 1-800-927-0176

(Available at your local drug store)
- Physicians Choice® Concealer Twins
- L'Oreal® Cover Expert Concealer
- For larger areas try Dermablend Body Cover Creme. To order call 877-900-6700.

• SPEED HEAL CUTS & WOUNDS

1. Keep wounds moist to prevent scarring and speed healing up to three times faster. Apply antibiotic ointment or petroleum jelly and cover with a bandage or liquid bandage to seal in moisture.

2. Burn and Wound Crème™ can help ease pain, contains stimulating vitamins and healing properties that promote new skin cell growth and speed recovery time. Every household should have Burn and Wound Crème in their First Aid Kit!

3. Allergic to antibiotic ointments? Tannins in black tea contract the skin, healing wounds quickly. Apply a wet tea bag on wounds for 10 to 15 minutes. Then apply petroleum jelly and cover with a bandage or liquid bandage.

4. Raw, unpasteurized honey contains natural antibacterial properties that can help heal wounds, infections, burns and prevent scarring. Apply raw honey then petroleum jelly and cover with a bandage if possible, or try Egyptian Magic All-

Purpose Healing Cream. It works wonders on burns and wounds. It contains bees wax, honey, olive oil, bee propollis and other healing ingredients. It's a top seller.

5. Apply Vitamin E or cocoa butter on wounds to keep them moist. Cover with a regular or liquid bandage to seal in moisture.

6. Zinc supplements can also aid in healing wounds.

BEST BEAUTY BUYS FOR CUTS & WOUNDS

(To order visit www.hollywoodbeautysecrets.com)
- Burn and Wound Crème™
- Egyptian Magic All-Purpose Healing Cream

(Available at your local drug store)
- Antibiotic Ointment
- New Skin™ Liquid Bandage
- Petroleum Jelly
- Palmer's Cocoa Butter® Formula with Vitamin E
- Vitamin E
- Zinc supplements

- **RELIEVING BURNS**

The following remedies can help burns. If you have a severe burn or have any sign of infection, see your doctor immediately.

1. Burn and Wound Crème™eases pain, minimizes blistering,

contains stimulating vitamins and healing properties that promote new skin cell growth and speed recovery time. Every household should have Burn and Wound Crème in their First Aid Kit.

2. Silvidine™ cream takes away heat and pain while rapidly healing burns. Treated areas turn the color black due to Silvidine's silver content. The black fades away after a few days. Damaged skin eventually peels. Firemen use Silvidine™. It is available by prescription.

3. Colloidal Silver can help heal burns and prevent infection. Vitamin C-Ester cream can help heal sun burns and reduces inflammation.

4. For sunburn, rubbing a tomato on skin can help provide some relief. Tomatoes contain Vitamin C and carotenoids which speed healing and can help relieve pain. Burn and wound cream can help relieve redness from sunburn.

5. Aloe vera gel contains allantoin which eases burns and speeds healing. Apply aloe gel several times a day and cover with gauze and a bandage.

6. Raw, unpasteurized honey helps heal minor burns and speeds healing with its natural antibiotic properties. Apply raw honey and cover with a bandage. Egyptian Magic All-Purposes Healing Cream also helps speed healing. It really works well.

7. Place a piece of raw potato on a burn for 10 minutes. The starchy juice containes enzymes and moisture to speed healing.

8. Onion contains healing properties. For a quick fix, apply a slice of onion to minor burns.

BEST BEAUTY BUYS FOR BURNS

Healing Products:

(To order visit www.hollywoodbeautysecrets.com)
- Burn and Wound Crème™
- Egyptian Magic All-Purpose Healing Cream
- Vitamin C-Ester cream by Derma e

(Available at your local health food store)
- Colloidal Silver by Wellness
- Raw honey
- Silvidine is available by prescription.

• SOOTHING HIVES

Hives can be triggered by a number of elements such as food, wine, bottled lemon juice (sulfites), allergies, medication, stress or hormonal changes. The release of the body's histamine causes red, itchy hives. The following remedies are known to help hives or provide temporary relief until you can see your doctor.

1. Apply witch hazel with a cotton pad. It instantly cools and soothes itching, reducing red bumps.

2. At night apply calamine lotion to itchy areas.

3. Pour one cup apple cider vinegar into warm tub water. Soak for 20 minutes. Then towel off. Do not rinse.

4. Add one box of corn starch to a large pot of hot water and

stir. Pour mixture into warm tub water. Soak for 20 minutes. Rinse with tepid water.

5. Drink 10 or more glasses of water per day. Add fresh lemon juice to water. *NOTE:* Do not use bottled lemon juice, as it often contains sulfites that can trigger hives.

6. Antihistamines such as Benadryl® or Zyrtec® can help ease hives as they block the production of histamine. Benadryl® is an effective over-the-counter medications. Zyrtec® requires a prescription. Check with your doctor before taking these antihistamines.

7. Strawberries, some nuts and red wines are common triggers. Have you had any of these lately?

BEST BEAUTY BUYS FOR HIVES

(Available at your local drug store)
- Benadryl®
- Witch Hazel
- Calamine Lotion
- Corn Starch
- Apple Cider Vinegar

• FADING BRUISES
These are some of the most effective remedies that can help fade bruises:

1. Saturate a cotton pad with witch hazel and apply to bruises.

2. To remedy bruises from the inside out the following supplements may help: Homeopathic Arnica Montana tablets, quercitine with bioflavinoids, horsetail, bromelaine, lecithin or grapeseed extract. Taking Rutin two to three months before surgery is known to help prevent severe bruising. Check with your doctor before taking these supplements.

3. Apply topical Arnica, Vitamin K Cream, Traumeel Gel, A-O-K Crème or creams containing Haloxyl to the bruised sights.

4. Taking vitamin C daily can help prevent and speed-heal bruises. Fruits and vegetables such as pineapple, green peas, red peppers, cantaloupe, strawberries and citrus fruits like oranges and tangerines are loaded with anti-bruise vitamins. Add a squirt of fresh lemon juice to drinking water.

BEST BEAUTY BUYS FOR FADING BRUISES

(Available at your local health food store)
- Witch Hazel
- Arnica Montana 30C
- The Rub (Arnica Cream) by NatraBio
- Traumeel® Anti-Inflammatory Cream or Ointment
- Grapeseed Extract by Natural Factors
- Vitamin K 7 Oils & 7 Herbs Crème by Orjene
- Rutin
- Bromelaine
- Quercitin

- **RELIEVING A HANGOVER**

ProEndorphin™ is loaded with B Vitamins. It is a mood booster and energizer that also relieves a hangover. Pour one packet into a glass of water and drink for quick relief.

BEST BEAUTY BUYS FOR A HANGOVER

(To order visit www.hollywoodbeautysecrets.com)
- ProEndorphin™

- **RELIEVING NAUSEA**

1. Ginger relieves nausea by reducing inflammation and neutralizing acid in the stomach.

2. Drink ginger tea. Boil a piece of gingerroot in a small pot of water. Let cool, remove ginger and drink tea.

3. Drink a glass of flat ginger ale. Keep an emergency six pack of ginger ale in the cupboard. If nausea persists, see your doctor.

BEST BEAUTY BUYS FOR NAUSEA
- Ginger root (in the produce section)
- Canada Dry Ginger Ale
- Diet Hansen's Ginger Ale

- **PREVENTING A COLD**

These effective remedies can help prevent a cold at the onset. Check with your doctor before taking supplements or remedies listed.

1. Drink 2 cups of green tea daily to boost immunity to colds, flu and some cancers. Polyphenols in the tea attach themselves to cells, preventing cold viruses and flu.

2. Taking Triphala daily can prevent colds. It contains antiviral properties.

3. Taking olive leaf at the onset of a cold can be beneficial. Olive leaf extract is an anti-bacterial, anti-viral and antifungal. Choose olive leaf extract containing 17% oleuropein.

4. At the onset of a cold insert Zicam ® homeopathic zinc gel into nostrils three times daily. Zicam® can help wipe out cold symptoms in three to four days. Add Triphala and/or olive leaf daily when feeling cold symptoms.

5. When around those with colds, rinse sinuses with saline nasal wash (saline and water solution) as soon as you get home. The rhinovirus starts in the nasal passages. By keeping nostrils clean you can prevent a cold. To prevent sickness when flying, rinse sinuses once you arrive at your destination.

6. Cold-EEZE® zinc tablets are clinically proven to quickly banish a cold.

7. Colds usually begin with a sore throat. Gargle with apple cider vinegar immediately to kill any bacteria. This will often prevent a cold. Gargling with salt-water is also effective.

BEST BEAUTY BUYS FOR PREVENTING A COLD

(Available at your local health food store)
- Green Tea
- Zicam®
- Ocean Nasal Spray
- Olive Leaf Extract by Solary
- Triphala by Solaray
- Cold-EEZE®
- Apple Cider Vinegar

- **RELIEVING A SORE THROAT**
1. Gargle with warm water and salt or a mouthful of apple cider vinegar. Listerine is also an effective gargle.

2. Take olive leaf extract and triphala at the onset of a sore throat. Olive leaf and triphala contain anti-viral and anti-bacterial properties.

3. Drink green tea daily to boost immunity to colds, flu, and even some cancers. Polyphenols (antioxidants) in the tea prevent viruses from attacking cells.

4. Red tea is naturally decaffeinated and loaded with antioxidants that fight disease. Drink it hot, iced, with lemon or milk. White tea has even more antioxidants.

5. Zinkers® sugar-free lemon zinc lozenges, relieve a sore throat and help fight a cold. Another good brand is Cold-EEZE®.

BEST BEAUTY BUYS FOR SORE THROAT RELIEF

(Available at your local health food store)
- Apple Cider Vinegar
- Zicam
- Cold-EEZE®
- Listerine
- Olive Leaf Extract by Solaray
- Triphala by Solaray
- Red Tea by Numi or Republic of Tea
- Zinker's ® Sugar-free Lemon Lozenges

Anti-Aging Alternatives

• ANTI-AGING FACTS

Americans are obsessed with perfection, youthful skin and staying slim. Social pressure to conform to standards of beauty and thinness explains why so many individuals are investing in rejuvenation and fat reducing technology such as high-tech lasers, injectables, anti-aging creams, fat-melting devices and weight loss books. Perhaps our fascination with rejuvenation is because the "baby boomer" is now the largest growing segment of our population. Americans are investing big bucks searching for the "Fountain of Youth." Just look at these recent facts:

- In 2001 Americans spent almost $3 billion dollars on anti-aging products.
- Studies reveal that when you feel attractive, you become more confident, accomplish more and will be more successful.
- On average, working women use more than 20 grooming products a day.
- In 2001, drug store chains reported over $19.2 billion dollars were spent on cosmetics alone.
- Botox™ stocks rose 60% just months after it was approved by the FDA.
- In 2001 over 5 million people altered their complexion using microdermabrasion or chemical peels.
- In 2002, over 40 billion dollars were spent on weight loss books.
- Firm, uplifted breasts symbolize youth. In the past five years breast lift procedures (mastopexies) have increased 203%.

Anti-Aging Alternatives

- According to The American Society for Aesthetic Plastic Surgery: 471% more non-surgical cosmetic procedures were performed in 2003 than six years ago and surgical cosmetic procedures have risen 87%.
- Men and even late teens are jumping on the cosmetic surgery bandwagon.

On a daily basis we are bombarded and fascinated with anti-aging procedures. You've likely seen Extreme Makeover and prime time television shows such as Dateline, 20/20, even news stations reporting the latest rejuvenation methods. They use 'teasers' to draw in millions of viewers - and they do!

The following treatments are effective, though slightly more costly anti-aging alternatives than those in the previous chapters. Concerns such as deep wrinkles, severe sun damage, sagging skin, pigmentation marks, melasma, rosacea, cellulite, acne scars, broken capillaries, spider veins, stretch marks and more are addressed in the following pages. If you have a particular area of concern, hopefully this information can help. Many cities in the United States provide these procedures. Ask your dermatologist for a referral or go to www.aboutskinsurgery.org to find a dermatologic surgeon in your area.

NOTE: *Please read this important note*. In the author's opinion, the following information is believed to be accurate. However, it is the reader's responsibility to extensively research and verify all information, procedures, doctor and facility credentials before proceeding with a treatment listed within these pages. The author, distributor and publisher disclaim any liability from use of procedures or information within these pages.

1. EXFOLIATING IS KEY TO YOUTHFUL SKIN

As mentioned earlier, the key secret to keeping skin youthful, firm and even in color is frequent exfoliation and protecting skin from the sun. Exfoliating helps smooth and loosen dull skin cells, evens skin tone, fades pigmentation spots, unclogs pores, stimulates collagen and elastin production and regenerates new skin cells more quickly. Avoiding sun exposure can prevent deep wrinkles and pigmentation spots.

When we are young skin cells naturally regenerate very quickly (about every 28 days). As we age skin cell regeneration slows down (about every 48 days). By exfoliating regularly you will speed cell regeneration similarly to when you were a child. The result is smooth, youthful, firm, even-colored, supple skin. Using baking soda or microdermabrasion-type scubs are highly effective choices. However, sometimes in special cases extra attention may be needed to help diminish deep wrinkles, severe sun damage, pigmentation spots and sagging skin.

Microdermabrasion Exfoliant

Microdermabrasion is an effective, fairly non-invasive way to help reduce fine lines, unclog pores, even out skin color and help fade discolorations. It is a non-surgical procedure that is performed by spraying a fine jet of mineral crystals onto the surface of the skin. As crystals are sprayed along the surface of the face, neck and chest, they are suctioned off along with dead surface skin cells. This technique is used for mild skin resurfacing. It is also effective for removing blackheads, whiteheads (clogged pores), smoothing stretch marks, rough, thick and dry skin, acne-prone skin and other minor scarring.

Because microdermabrasion exfoliates the skin, it stimulates collagen and elastin production. To achieve effective results a series of treatments is recommended. You will most likely be given a skin lightening or retinoid cream to apply between sessions if pigmentation or wrinkles are your primary concern. Side effects: a little redness. There is no down time or healing time required. In fact, many celebrities and models have the procedure done the day before an important event like the Oscars, Emmy's, other award shows or photo shoots. It gives the face a beautiful glow! Microdermabrasion is considered a 'lunch time' facial. It can be safely performed on all skin types. On a budget? Try the Microdermabrasion Scrub described at the beginning of the book or simply use baking soda if you have normal, dry mature or oily skin that is not sensitive. Do not use Microdermabrasion if you have rosacea.

Resources:
- Marina del Rey, CA. Sue Sigrist, 310-822-8873.
- Marina del Rey, CA. The Skin Rejuvenation and Laser Medical Center, CA. 310-306-7100. Mention this book to receive a 10% discount.
- Santa Monica, CA. Dr. Ava Shamban, 310-828-2282
- Torrance, CA. Dr. David M.Duffy, 310-370-5679

(To order visit www.hollywoodbeautysecrets.com)
- Microdermabrasion Scrub

2. DIMINISHING PIGMENTATION SPOTS
L.E.D. Light Therapy

L.E.D. Light Therapy can help dramatically fade pigmentation spots while at the same time take years off your face by diminishing fine lines and preventing wrinkles. Anti-aging, affordable, non-invasive and painless L.E.D. therapy could likely replace costly, painful laser resurfacing and face-lift surgery. It's scientifically and clinically documented to stimulate collagen, help diminish brown or red spots, rosacea, smooth texture, reduce blemishes, form new capillaries, increase circulation, help repair and even prevent wrinkles. It can also help relieve pain, arthritis pain and age spots from hands. You'll be hearing more about L.E.D. Light Therapy in the next few years. L.E.D. Light Therapy is totally safe and can be used on ANY skin color, or any age skin. L.E.D. Light Therapy emits wavelengths of warm light that help the body's ability to repair tissue. It has been used by both NASA and the US Army to help quickly heal broken bones, sprains, wounds and more. Athletes have been privy to L.E.D. light therapy to quickly heal their injuries. Its proven anti-aging benefits have also been clinically documented. Many celebrities have purchased costly salon units for personal use at about $9,000. Salon treatments vary from $65 to $125 per session. However, powerful home units are much more cost effective and are now available. Read more about L.E.D. Light Therapy at the beginning of the book.

Resources:
L.E.D. Light Therapy:

- Redlands, CA. Aesthetic Skin Care, 909-798-6766
- Fountain Valley, CA. Dr. E. Llorente, 714-885-8980
- Encino, CA. Epic The Salon, 818-716-8851
- Connecticut, Anna Lamorte, 203-778-2858
- Honolulu, HI. Wellness Institute, 808-941-6300
- Washington, Studio Donna Spa, 425-258-4941
- New Jersey, Katherine's Aesthetics, 201-802-9300

To order a home unit email louisa@hollywoodbeautysecrets.com or call 1-877-568-4727.

Micro-Current

This completely non-invasive, anti-aging treatment has been used by NASA and Hollywood celebrities for years. Nature and technology with micro-current helps diminish pigmentation spots as well as helps repair cells and tissue, stimulates collagen, elastin, increases muscle tone, helps repair deep lines, wrinkles, scars, and rosacea. I can't name names but you'd be surprised at the Who's Who list using this secret weapon for anti-aging and diminishing age spots. Micro-Current can also help diminish cellulite, detoxify the body, heal bruising and wounds. It has even been used to treat some diseases. It's also reasonably priced.

Resources:
* F. Perez, Santa Monica, CA. 310-899-6807

IPL Photofacial:

IPL (Intense Pulsed Light), Photorejuvenation or Photofacial can help fade freckles, pigmentation spots, sun damage, rosacea, broken capillaries, port wine stains, birthmarks, dilated blood vessels and help diminish fine lines. It can also refine enlarged pores, tighten and tone skin. IPL is not a laser. Intense light energy heats as it penetrates through the skin's surface down to the collagen, without damaging or burning surface skin. IPL requires numbing cream prior to treatment as the light feels like a snap of a rubber band. NOTE: IPL cannot be performed on skin of color. This procedure can dramatically reduce the redness associated with rosacea and port wine stains. It also stimulates the production of collagen and elastin, creating more youthful-looking, toned, smooth skin. IPL Photofacial is non-invasive and considered a 'lunch time' facial though there is a little down time due to darkened spots. Freckles or pigmentation spots darken for an approx. seven to 10 days, then flake off or become absorbed by the body. Depending on the condition you are treating, four to six sessions may be required. It is somewhat costly ranging from $250 to $550 a session. Stay out of the sun before an IPL treatment.

Resources:
- Marina del Rey, CA. The Skin Rejuvenation and Laser Medical Center, 310-306-7100 Mention this book to receive a 10% discount.
- Santa Monica, CA. Dr. Ava Shamban, 310-828-2282
- Torrance, CA. Dr. David M. Duffy, 310-370-5679

3. MINIMALLY INVASIVE FACELIFTS AND DIMINISHING WRINKLES

L.E.D. Light Therapy

Take years off your face with affordable L.E.D. Light Therapy. Anti-aging, non-invasive and painless light therapy could likely replace costly, painful laser resurfacing and face-lift surgery. It's scientifically and clinically documented to stimulate collagen, help diminish brown or red spots, rosacea, smooth texture, reduce blemishes, form new capillaries, increase circulation, help repair and even prevent wrinkles. You'll be hearing more about L.E.D. Light Therapy in the next few years. L.E.D. Light Therapy is totally safe and can be used on ANY skin color, or any age skin. L.E.D. lights emit wavelengths of warm light that help the body's ability to repair tissue. It has been used by both NASA and the US Army to help quickly heal broken bones, sprains, wounds and more. Athletes have been privy to light therapy to quickly heal their injuries. Its proven anti-aging benefits have also been clinically documented. AND it's affordable! Super Bright LED bulbs deliver warm, non-invasive heat which penetrates into the skin to stimulate the production of collagen, thus repairing and reducing the formation of wrinkles and can help prevent sagging skin. An increase of blood flow to the skin improves the skin tone and texture. Skin tightens and firms, pores become more refined, uneven skin diminishes. You'll notice broken capillaries diminishing, age spots fading, wrinkles smoothing and skin tightening in just six to eight treatments (sometimes even less). After just one treatment, rosacea flush can diminish. After six to eight treatments you'll need only one treatment a month for maintenance, however, you can't overuse L.E.D. Light Therapy. Apply the unit on the tops of the hands to help diminish age spots! So many benefits. It can even help relieve joint and back pain.

L.E.D. Light Therapy is most effective when combined with exfoliation. Simply exfoliate face with Microdermabrasion Scrub or baking soda prior to L.E.D. Light Therapy so heat and light can better penetrate. Combine L.E.D. Light Therapy with skin care products containing Matrixyl or antioxidant-rich creams or serums for even more effective rejuvenating results. For more information email louisa@hollywoodbeautysecrets.com

Resources:
L.E.D. Light Therapy:
To order home unit email louisa@hollywoodbeautysecrets.com or call 1-877-568-4727.
- Redlands, CA. Aesthetic Skin Care, 909-798-6766
- Fountain Valley, CA. Dr. E. Llorente, 714-885-8980
- Encino, CA. Epic The Salon, 818-716-8851
- Connecticut, Anna Lamorte, 203-778-2858
- Honolulu, HI. Wellness Institute, 808-941-6300

- Washington, Studio Donna Spa, 425-258-4941
- New Jersey, Katherine's Aesthetics, 201-802-9300

elos™ Polaris & Galaxy Wrinkle Treatment

Revolutionary elos™ uses bi-polar radio frequency combined with light energy to significantly help reduce the signs of aging. Results may even be equivalent to laser resurfacing with no down time. Matrix heating works at both the deep dermis and surface of the skin treating both fine and deep wrinkles. The procedure takes approximately one hour to perform. Numbing cream is applied and the procedure is performed using a Zimmer™ Chiller to cool the skin, helping to reduce discomfort. Make-up can be applied immediately afterward. Some individuals may experience temporary swelling for 24 hours and redness which subsides within an hour. Many practitioners charge $1000 per session. The Redlands location listed below charges only $650 per session. One practitioner states that this treatment has shown superior results over Radio Frequency (mono-polar) treatments alone.

Resources:
- Redlands, CA. Aesthetic Skin Care Toll Free, 866-368-SKIN or 909-798-6796

Micro-Current

This completely non-invasive, anti-aging treatment has been used by NASA and Hollywood celebrities for decades. Nature and technology with micro-current helps repair cells and tissue, stimulates collagen, elastin, increases muscle tone, helps repair deep lines, wrinkles, scars, pigmentation spots and rosacea. I can't name names but you'd be surprised at the Who's Who list using this secret weapon for anti-aging. It's also reasonably priced.

Resources:
- F. Perez, Santa Monica, CA. 310-899-6807

4. CHEMICAL PEELS

Chemical peels are generally for resurfacing skin, treating deep lines, severe sun damage, freckles, pigmentation spots and smoothing pock-marked skin. A chemical peel may be something you are considering. However, before you make up your mind, be sure to review the extensive list of affordable non-invasive options listed in this section.

Chemical peels would not be my first recommendation to anyone as they can be, for the most part, extremely invasive. However, one popular and less invasive chemical peel is the beta salicylic acid peel. It can be used on all skin types including skin of color. If you are considering a chemical peel, choose a dermatologist or professional aesthetician who is highly experienced with chemical peels as inexperience can cause severely burned or scarred skin. This is your face we're talking about! For skin of color, see the paragraph below.

Beta Salicylic Acid Peel For All Skin Types

Beta Salicylic Acid peels are safe for all skin types including skin of color. BSA peels self-neutralize and do not burn out of control like other types of peels. After the BSA peel skin will become dry and tight with light peeling, random white flakes or exfoliation for one to two days. Remember to apply sunscreen each and every day to protect your new, even and smooth complexion.

Part Twelve

Note to Those With Skin of Color

Those with skin of color, particularly darker black women, should avoid chemical peels such as alpha hydroxy acid, TCA and Phenol Peels or dermabrasion as they can frequently cause burned or hyper-pigmented skin. However, Beta Salicylic Acid peels in concentrations up to 20%, can be safe. Darker black women do well with this peel provided they follow a four-week protocol prior to the treatment. Otherwise hyper-pigmentation may occur. Avoid going to a facility or practitioner who says it's okay to do the BSA peel without the bleaching protocol or you may risk severe skin damage.

Pre-Peel Protocol For Skin of Color:

For the best possible results, those with skin of color should follow this protocol. A minimum of four weeks prior to the beta salicylic acid peel treatment apply a prescription bleaching cream nightly. It consists of a mix of hydroquinone, kojic acid and retinoic acid. This effective bleaching cream will be provided by the practitioner and must be applied each and every night for a minimum of four weeks. Then every morning, you will need to apply an SPF 30 or stronger sunscreen (see next paragraph for effective sunscreen suggestions). This pre-peel protocol causes the melanin-producing cells to go dormant, exfoliates skin, refines the pores, induces collagen formation, produces tighter and firmer skin, decreases fine lines and wrinkles as well as evens skin tone. Sunscreen should be worn each and every day after the treatment is performed to maintain the results.

Post-Peel Protocol For ALL Skin Types:

Protect your sensitive, smooth and newly-even skin from the sun after having a chemical peel. Wear a visor and an SPF 30 sunscreen each and every day. For complete protection choose sunscreen that contains one of the following effective UV protectant ingredients: zinc oxide, titanium dioxide, Parsol® or avobenzene.

Other Types of Chemical Peels

Customized chemical peels like Jessner, Carbolic, or Glycolic acid (AHA of 40% or higher concentration) can help reduce fine lines, stimulate collagen and elastin production which firms skin, and can help smooth and even skin tones. You may feel a hot, tingly sensation with some chemical peel treatments. These are not recommended for skin of color.

Deeper peels require topical anesthetic, followed by dressings and/or ointments for a few days. You may experience swelling, blisters, redness, oozing or peeling which can last up to two weeks. Skin may be pink for several weeks so wearing sun block is extremely important. Milder chemical peels are under 40% glycolic acid concentrations and can cause red or irritated skin for approximately one week. Stronger concentrations (50% to 70% glycolic acid) may cause oozing, red skin and peeling for up to four weeks.

Resources:
- Redlands, CA. Aesthetic Skin Care Toll Free, 866-368-SKIN (ask about their 5 step peel for only $85)
- Santa Monica, CA. Dr. Ava Shamban, 310-828-2282
- Torrance, CA. Dr. David M. Duffy, 310-370-5679

- Marina del Rey, CA. Medical Aesthetician Sue Sigrist, 310-301-0363

5. LASER UPDATE

Laser resurfacing can still be somewhat invasive, however, there are a few new non-invasive laser treatment options that may be of interest. Because lasers can be controlled precisely, the risk of complications and scarring is minimal. Laser is a bloodless procedure that heat-seals blood vessels. Lasers can smooth wrinkles considerably, even out color and texture of skin, diminish acne scars, port wine stains, birthmarks, growths and spider veins. Lasers generate electrons. Lasers use organic solid or liquid dye, gas, light or radio frequency. Some lasers are more invasive than others. Here is an explanation several types of lasers available:

- Pulse-dye lasers treat dilated blood vessels, veins and port wine stains. They vaporize pigment on the surface of the skin without bleeding.
- Co2 lasers are used for skin rejuvenation and treating deep wrinkles as they penetrate more deeply into the skin. They tighten the skin which may prevent the need for a facelift. Side effects: may cause up to 6 months of redness.
- SmoothBeam™ Laser is an alternative to Co2 lasers. It stimulates collagen production and can reduce up to 75% of wrinkles.
- Diode lasers use infrared light to treat dilated blood vessels, brown spots, freckles and permanently remove hair.

Lasers for Skin of Color

For skin of color (African-American, Hispanic or Asian) some lasers may cause uneven pigmentation. Recommended lasers for skin of color are: YAG (Nd:YAG); diode; ruby; KTP; and non-ablative lasers. The diode is particularly beneficial for removing the small black mole-like growths which are commonly seen on the face and neck area in Asian and African-American individuals. YAG (Nd:YAG); diode; ruby; KTP; and non-ablative lasers help refine texture, fine lines, skin tone and even out scars successfully. After some laser procedures the skin may ooze or become red and flaky. See an experienced dermatologist or laser specialist.

Resources:

- Redlands, CA. Aesthetic Skin Care Toll Free, 866-368-SKIN (ask about their 5 step peel for only $85)
- Santa Monica, CA. Dr. Ava Shamban, 310-828-2282
- Torrance, CA. Dr. David M. Duffy, 310-370-5679
- Beverly Hills, CA. Smoothbeam™, Epione Center
- Marina del Rey, CA. The Skin Rejuvenation and Laser Medical Center, 310-306-7100. Mention this book to receive a 10% discount.

6. WRINKLE FILLERS OR INJECTABLES

Many types of injectable substances can fill in wrinkles, sunken areas of the face, expression lines, small imperfections and scars. These are the latest fillers, implants and injectables available:

Bovine Collagen Injections

Collagen keeps our skin firm and youthful looking. As we age, however, collagen production slows down and elastin fibers break down resulting in wrinkles. Exfoliating stimulates collagen production and collagen can also be injected into the skin for quick, effective results. Approved by the FDA for the past 17 years, bovine collagen is injected into the skin to smooth wrinkles, plump up sunken areas of the face and fill in scars or pock marks. Redness, swelling, stinging, throbbing or bruising may occur at the injection sites. Within a week the redness and bruising should disappear. Stinging and throbbing stops within hours. Allergic reactions are rare but can occur with bovine collagen. A skin test is done prior to being treated. Itching or stiffness at the injection site can occur but is rare. Apply numbing cream one hour before treatment as collagen injections can be somewhat painful. Because collagen is eventually absorbed by the body, the effects are temporary, lasting about two to six months. Collagen is not recommended for pregnant women, those who have beef allergies or who suffer from auto-immune diseases.

Human Grade Collagen Injections

CosmoPlast® and CosmoDerm® are FDA approved human collagen fillers. Unlike bovine collagen they do not require an allergy test.

Resources:

- Redlands, CA. Aesthetic Skin Care Toll Free, 866-368-SKIN
- Marina del Rey, CA. Contact The Skin Rejuvenation and Laser Medical Center, 310-306-7100. Mention this book and receive a 10% discount.
- Torrance, CA. Contact Dr. David M. Duffy, 310-370-5679

Restylane®

Restylane® is a clear gel filler derived from hyaluronic acid which naturally occurs in the body. The gel is called Non-Animal Stabilized Hyaluronic Acid. It is biodegradable and eliminates any risk of allergic reaction. Restylane adds fullness to folds or wrinkles and is known to last longer than collagen (approx. eight months). A numbing gel or nerve blocker is used for injecting lips. Do not take aspirin, Vitamin E and St. John's Worth prior to injections. Side effects: cold sores may be exacerbated and some women report experiencing small bumps or lumps.

Resources:
* Fountain Valley, CA. Dr. E. Llorente, (714) 885-8980
* Redlands, CA. Aesthetic Skin Care Toll Free, 866-368-SKIN

Fat Injections

Fat injections and fat transplanting are becoming increasingly more popular than collagen and may replace the need for a face-lift. Sagging skin, hollowed areas including cheeks, neck and under eyes occur as we age and collagen stimulation slows down. By injecting fat in the hollowed areas, one can look years younger. It's quite safe and far less invasive or costly than a face-lift. The fat is taken from your own tummy, buttocks or thighs using a large-bore needle. The advantage of using your own fat is that there are no allergic reactions. Its effects are the same as collagen - plumping up wrinkles, lines and scars. Overfilling the site is necessary as it takes a few weeks for the fat to absorb. The injection sites may look a little swollen for a few days. The body will eventually absorb the fat over time so re-injecting will be required.

Botox™

FDA-approved Botox™ is a very popular and effective purified protein and paralyzing neurotoxin. It is injected into specific muscles of the face causing temporary paralysis so expression and frown lines are banished. It does not travel into other areas of the body. You will experience stinging while it is being injected. Bruising may likely also occur. Ice the area before injections. Some doctors have cooling machines which they direct onto the site before injecting to eliminate bruising. Many doctors are now using smaller needles in order to prevent bruising. To save money and prevent looking too stiff, consider injecting just a few areas of the face such as the frown lines between the eyes and just a few injections in the forehead so you have a more natural look. The effects last approximately three months. Botox™ must be used within a four hour period of opening the vial or it loses its potency. Be leery of low prices as you may be getting a diluted or stale batch. If the effects of Botox™ do not last three months, insist on a discount on your next visit. Beware of Botox™ parties.

Resources:
- Fountain Valley, CA. Dr. E. Llorente, (714) 885-8980
- Redlands, CA. Aesthetic Skin Care Toll Free, 866-368-SKIN
- Marina del Rey, CA. Dr. Abraham Tzadik, 310-305-1020. Mention this book to receive a 10% discount
- Marina del Rey, CA. The Skin Rejuvenation and Laser Medical Center, 310-306-7100. Mention this book to receive a 10% discount on Botox™
- Go to www.aboutskinsurgery.org for local contacts.

7. RELIEVING ACNE
Micro Peel

The Micro Peel is a three-step 20-minute peel that removes the top layer of skin. It is used to treat sun-damage, uneven pigmentation or acne-prone skin. It is not used for reducing wrinkles. An enzyme peel is applied to exfoliate the skin. Then a 15-30% concentration alpha hydroxy acid solution is applied for about two minutes. Lastly, the skin is cooled using cryogenic (cooling) therapy. The result is refined pores, uniform color, sun-damaged skin is repaired, pores become unblocked and skin is smooth. Monthly or bimonthly treatments are recommended.

SmoothBeam™

FDA-approved SmoothBeam™ laser is a highly effective treatment that helps clear acne and smoothes skin. It works by heating the oil glands reducing oil production. It involves a cool spray on the surface of the skin while the heat of the laser attacks the sebaceous glands where oil is produced. SmoothBeam™ diminishes acne scars by creating mild injury to the dermis. This stimulates collagen production beneath the surface and smoothes the top layer of the skin. Skin may become pink for up to two hours afterwards. Treatments can be painful. Talk to your physician or dermatologist about this highly effective laser treatment.

Blue Light Therapy

Blue Light Therapy uses cold light to help diminish acne. It helps stop the production of sebum in pores, thus helps prevent and relieves acne. For skin of color, Blue Light Therapy combined with a beta salicylic acid peel, can help improve acne-prone or pock-marked. Beyond CP Lotion applied daily after treatments and each day helps keeps blemishes and acne in check.

Practitioners who perform Red Light Therapy for anti-aging will likely also have Blue Light Therapy as professional units are equipped with both lights. Blue Light Therapy home units are now available. For more information email louisa@hollywoodbeautysecrets.com.

Resources:
- Redlands, CA. Aesthetic Skin Care 909-798-6766
- Fountain Valley, CA. Dr. E. Llorente, 714-885-8980
- Encino, CA. Epic The Salon, 818-716-8851
- Connecticut, Anna Lamorte, 203-778-2858
- Honolulu, HI. Wellness Institute, 808-941-6300
- Washington, Studio Donna Spa, 425-258-4941
- New Jersey, Katherine's Aesthetics, 201-802-9300

Clear Light™

Clear Light, a high-intensity light treatment, attacks the bacteria that causes acne. This treatment is highly beneficial to those who cannot tolerate antibiotics or the side effects associated with acne prescriptions. In four weeks acne will clear. Clear Light can be used on all areas of the body. Talk to your physician or dermatologist about this highly effective light therapy.

Resources:
- Beverly Hills, CA. Beverly Hills Laser & Rejuvenation Medical Group, Inc.,1-800-282-4555 (Clear Light)
- Beverly Hills, CA. Epione, 310-271-6506 SmoothBeam™
- Go to www.biomedic.com for MicroPeel.
- Go to www.aboutskinsurgery.org for local contacts.

8. SPIDER AND VARICOSE VEINS
Sclerotherapy
Sclerotherapy can help diminish both spider and varicose veins. A solution is injected into the veins causing them to collapse and lighten in color. The body absorbs the vein over the course of a few weeks. Sclerotherapy can also be performed on hands to diminish aging veins. See an experienced phlebologist. There is some down time.

Resources:
- Torrance, CA. Dr. David Duffy, 310-370-5679
- Redlands, CA. Aesthetic Skin Care Toll Free 866-368-SKIN
- Fountain Valley, CA. Dr. E. Llorente, 714-885-8980

Irodex™ Diode Laser
The Irodex™Diode laser is an extremely powerful and effective method of diminishing spider veins - virtually eliminating them.

Resources:
Irodex Diode Laser & Sclerotherapy:
- Redlands, CA. Aesthetic Skin Care, 909-798-6766
- Torrance, CA. Dr. D. Duffy, 310-370-5679

elos™ Polaris & Galaxy Wrinkle Treatment
Revolutionary elos™ uses bi-polar radio frequency combined with light energy to significantly help reduce spider veins and broken capillaries. Matrix heating works at both the deep dermis and surface. The procedure takes approximately one hour to perform. Numbing cream is applied and the procedure is performed using a Zimmer™ Chiller to cool the skin, which helps reduce discomfort. Avoid extreme heat or exercise for 24

hours. Some individuals may experience temporary swelling for 24 hours and/or redness which subsides within an hour.

Resources:
- Redlands, CA. Aesthetic Skin Care Toll Free, 866-368-SKIN

VascuLight™ & Nd:YAG™Lasers

VascuLight ™and Nd: YAG lasers heat and destroy spider veins. A topical numbing cream is applied for comfort. The veins are eventually absorbed by the body. Keep the treated areas out of the sun both before and after treatment for several weeks. Three or more sessions may be required.

Resources:

- Marina del Rey, CA. The Skin Rejuvenation and Laser Medical Center, 310-306-7100. Mention this book to receive a 10% discount.
- Torrance, CA. Dr. D. Duffy, 310-370-5679
- Santa Monica, CA. Dr. Ava Shamban, 310-828-2282

Telangitron ®

The Telangitron® delivers low levels of high frequency and galvanic currents that coagulate the red blood vessels. A tiny needle, like those used for acupuncture, targets the blood vessels. You'll achieve immediate, results without scarring the surrounding tissue or creating any down time. Depending on the number of vessels, you will see immediate results. Numbing cream is applied pre-treatment. Dermatologists, laser and vein clinics and licensed aestheticians in some US states are trained to do this treatment. See resources below for practitioners.

Resources:
Telagangitron™
- Santa Barbara, CA. Mike Bono, 805-682-4627
- Long Beach, CA. Dr. Cary Feibleman, 562-595-4777
- Fairfax, VA. Dr. Kevin Scott, 703-620-4300
- New Paltz, NY. Dr. Steven Weinman, 845-255-1919
- Lafayette, LA. Dr. K. Odinet, 337-233-0244
- For Telangitron™ practitioners in your area call 800-603-4996

9. BROKEN CAPILLARIES, ANGIOMA AND TELANGIECTASIA

To help diminish broken capillaries, angioma, skin tags, and telangiectasia (red-nose syndrome), the Telangitron® is highly effective. Telangiectasia on the upper body and face are caused by sun damage, age or they're inherited. This treatment delivers low levels of high frequency and galvanic currents for immediate results without scarring the surrounding tissue. There is no down time either. It is a non-invasive and affordable treatment. Dermatologists, laser and vein clinics and licensed aestheticians in some US states are trained to do this treatment.

Resources:
Telagangitron™
- Santa Barbara, CA Mike Bono, 805-682-4627
- Long Beach, CA. Dr. Cary Feibleman, 562-595-4777
- Fairfax, VA. Dr. Kevin Scott, 703-620-4300
- New Paltz, NY. Dr. Steven Weinman, 845-255-1919
- Lafayette, LA Dr. K. Odinet, 337-233-0244
- For Telangitron™practitioners in your area call 800-603-4996

10. DIMINISHING STRETCH MARKS
Intense Pulsed Light (IPL)

Intense Pulsed Light (IPL) can help diminish both red and blue stretch marks. It does not diminish older, white stretch marks as IPL senses only dark pigments. IPL is FDA approved. Consider applying topical Scar Gel to help diminish stretch marks. Available at www.hollywoodbeautysecrets.com.

ReLume™

ReLume ultra violet light stimulates the melanin production in skin to create pigmentation. This diminishes white stretch marks. Six or more treatments are usually required. ReLume is FDA-approved.

CoolBeam™

CoolBeam utilizes a Nd:YAG laser to return red, purple and white stretch marks to normal skin color. Results can be seen after three to six sessions. CoolBeam™ will not restore the smoothness of skin. Apply StriVectin SD cream to help smooth skin.

Resources:
- Torrance, CA. Dr. David M. Duffy, 310-370-5679
- Santa Monica, CA. Dr. Ava Shamban, 310-828-2282
- Beverly Hills, CA. Epion 310-271-6506
- Go to www.aboutskinsurgery.org for local practitioners

Permanent Make-Up for Stretch Marks

Permanent make-up can be injected into white stretch marks to even skin tone.

Resources:
- Society of Permanent Cosmetic Professionals (SPCP)
  888-584-SPCP www.spcp.org/memberlist.html
- Marina del Rey, CA. Aesthetician Lillia Svartsman
  (permanent make-up) 310-577-1077.
- Fountain Valley, CA. Tracy Watson P.M.E.
  714-885-8980

11. FAT INSTEAD OF A FACELIFT

"Pulling the face back is not the answer to aging skin. I think that plastic surgeons may have it wrong," admits a prominent plastic surgeon. He went on to explain that face-lifts are not the answer to aging, sagging skin. He explained that a simple and highly effective procedure which is very popular is injecting the face, neck and hands with fat. As we age our collagen, elastin, hyaluronic acid and human growth hormone production slows down. The result is sagging, hollowed areas of the face and neck and bony fingers.

Injecting fat into the hollowed areas of the face, neck and around the bony tendons of the hands can be a quicker, less costly way to achieve a more youthful-looking appearance. Fat injections are more effective, less invasive and far less costly than traditional plastic surgery.

Resources:
- Hollywood, CA. , Dr. G Ablon, Raleigh Studios

12. TREATMENT FOR YOUTHFUL-LOOKING HANDS

Brown spots, protruding veins and bony fingers are associated with aged-looking hands. Carrying heavy items creates blood to pool into the veins of the hands and will create protruding veins over time. L.E.D. Light Therapy can stimulate collagen and help diminish brown spots on hands. It also helps reduce arthritis pain which can cripple and may even eventually disfigure the hands. Sclerotherapy can also be used for hand rejuvenation. Dr. D. Duffy is a pioneer of sclerotherapy for the hands. Injecting fat around the tendons of the hands can also help rejuvenate the look of hands.

Resources:

L.E.D. Light Therapy:
- Fountain Valley, CA., Dr. E. Llorente 714-885-8980
- Redlands, CA. Aesthetic Skin Care Toll Free, 866-368-SKIN

Fat Injections:
- Hollywood, CA., Dr. G. Ablon, Raleigh Studios
- Redlands, CA. Aesthetic Skin Care Toll Free, 866-368-SKIN

Sclerotherapy:
- Torrance, CA. Dr. David Duffy, 310-370-5670 or 310-370-5679
- Santa Monica, CA. Dr. Ava Shamban, 310-828-2282
- Redlands, CA. Aesthetic Skin Care Toll Free, 866-368-SKIN

13. A NOTE ABOUT COSMETIC SURGERY

There are two types of surgeons who perform cosmetic surgery; plastic surgeons and cosmetic surgeons. A plastic surgeon is trained to perform plastic surgery for a period of four to five years and is board certified by the American Board of Plastic surgery. A cosmetic surgeon is an M.D. who has taken training to perform various plastic surgery procedures but has not had the four to five years specialty training in plastic surgery. Keep in mind that a competent plastic or cosmetic surgeon will only perform a "natural" looking procedure. When choosing a surgeon arrange to meet some patients who've had the procedure you would like. View "before" and "after" pictures. Ask the doctor if he/she has ever been sued. This is a legitimate question. Should the doctor react adversely, walk out the door. If his or her staff has had any of the procedures, they are happy with their results and they look natural, it is a good indication of the result you'll get. *NOTE:* You will rarely see a highly regarded plastic or cosmetic surgeon advertising. His/her reputation is usually word-of-mouth.

14. PERMANENT HAIR REMOVAL

Diode LightSheer™ can be used on a wide range of skin types. However, burning of the skin, a rare but occasional side effect, is less likely to occur with the newer Palomar SPL 1000. It was designed for use on darker skinned individuals such as Asians, Hispanics and African-Americans. Apply topical numbing cream one hour before the procedure. For under arms, legs, back and bikini line, repeat treatment every four to six weeks for a total of six to eight visits. For facial hair repeat treatment every four weeks. Facial hair grows more quickly than body hair.

Resources:
- Brentwood, CA. Launa Stone, R.N., 310-820-9761. Mention this book to receive a 10% discount.
- Marina del Rey, CA. The Skin Rejuvenation and Laser Medical Center, 310-306-7100. Palomar SLP 1000 and Diode LightSheer ™ are available at this location.
- Redlands, CA. Aesthetic Skin Care, 909-798-6766

15. PERMANENT COSMETIC MAKE-UP

Permanent make-up (Intradermal Pigmentation) can be a completely safe procedure when performed by a competent, experienced practitioner. Natural pigments are inserted into the dermal layer of the skin to fill in sparse brows, balance the shape of lips, darken lip color, line eyes, enhance hairline, restore areola, reduce the look of stretch marks and camouflage scars. *NOTE:* Choose an experienced permanent make-up technician, preferably also an artist. Get referrals. See "before" and "after" photos of previous clients. Ask if you can speak to or meet previous clients. Bring a friend for a second opinion on shape and color when doing brows. Numbing cream is applied during the procedure.

Resources:

- Society of Permanent Cosmetic Professionals (SPCP) 888-584-SPCP www.spcp.org/memberlist.html
- Marina del Rey, CA. Aesthetician Lillia Svartsman (permanent make-up) 310-577-1077.
- Fountain Valley, CA. Tracy Watson P.M.E. 714-885-8980

HollywoodBeautySecrets
P.O.Box 10692, Marina del Rey, CA 90295
Phone: 1-877-LOUISAS (568-4727)

Loyalty Discount Order Form

Hollywood Beauty Secrets Book	**13.95**
Microdermabrasion Scrub	**29.95**
Relastyl™	**56.95**
Perfect RX Nite Serum	**63.00**
DMAE Retexturizing Crème	**19.95**
Age Reversal Hand Crème	**16.50**
Ultimate Eye Crème	**39.95**
Aging Eraser	**47.95**
Acne & Scar Crème	**39.95**
Astazanthin & Pycnogenol Crème	**37.95**
High Potency Vit. C Serum	**44.95**
JoinTastik	**39.95**
Aloe Seltzer C	**26.00**
Under 30-Minute Model Sculpting Workout	**12.95**

Method of Payment:
Sorry, no personaly checks. Cashier's Checks or Money orders only.

Visa ( ) Mastercard ( ) Amex ( ) Discover ( )

___|___|___|___|___|___|___|___|___|___|___|___|___|___|___|____

Expiration Date: _____/_____

Signature: _____

Name: _____daytime phone # _____

Address: _____

City: _____ Zip _____ State _____

CA residents please add 8.25% sales tax.

S & H fees: : $5.95 for order total up to $19.99, $7.50 for order total up to $59.99, $10.00 for order total up to $99.99, $12.50 for order total up to $149.99, $16.50 for order total up to $249.99. Free shipping for orders $250+.

For fun, affordable, quality lingerie, visit
www.lingerieperfetta.com
Receive 10% off when you mention Hollywood Beauty Secrets!

HollywoodBeautySecrets
P.O.Box 10692, Marina del Rey, CA 90295
Phone: 1-877-LOUISAS (568-4727)

Loyalty Discount Order Form

Hollywood Beauty Secrets Book	13.95
Microdermabrasion Scrub	29.95
Relastyl™	56.95
Perfect RX Nite Serum	63.00
DMAE Retexturizing Crème	19.95
Age Reversal Hand Crème	16.50
Ultimate Eye Crème	39.95
Aging Eraser	47.95
Acne & Scar Crème	39.95
Astazanthin & Pycnogenol Crème	37.95
High Potency Vit. C Serum	44.95
JoinTastik	39.95
Aloe Seltzer C	26.00
Under 30-Minute Model Sculpting Workout	12.95

Method of Payment :
Sorry, no personaly checks. Cashier's Checks or Money orders only.

Visa ( ) Mastercard ( ) Amex ( ) Discover ( )
__|__|__|__|__|__|__|__|__|__|__|__|__|__|__|__
Expiration Date: _____/_____
Signature: _____
Name: _____daytime phone # _____
Address: _____
City: _____ Zip _____ State _____
CA residents please add 8.25% sales tax.
S & H fees: : $5.95 for order total up to $19.99, $7.50 for order total up to $59.99, $10.00 for order total up to $99.99, $12.50 for order total up to $149.99, $16.50 for order total up to $249.99. Free shipping for orders $250+.

For fun, affordable, quality lingerie, visit
www.lingerieperfetta.com
Receive 10% off when you mention Hollywood Beauty Secrets!

HollywoodBeautySecrets
P.O.Box 10692, Marina del Rey, CA 90295
Phone: 1-877-LOUISAS (568-4727)

Loyalty Discount Order Form

Hollywood Beauty Secrets Book	13.95
Microdermabrasion Scrub	29.95
Relastyl™	56.95
Perfect RX Nite Serum	63.00
DMAE Retexturizing Crème	19.95
Age Reversal Hand Crème	16.50
Ultimate Eye Crème	39.95
Aging Eraser	47.95
Acne & Scar Crème	39.95
Astazanthin & Pycnogenol Crème	37.95
High Potency Vit. C Serum	44.95
JoinTastik	39.95
Aloe Seltzer C	26.00
Under 30-Minute Model Sculpting Workout	12.95

Method of Payment :
Sorry, no personaly checks. Cashier's Checks or Money orders only.

Visa ( ) Mastercard ( ) Amex ( ) Discover ( )

___|___|___|___|___|___|___|___|___|___|___|___|___|___|___|___

Expiration Date: _____/_____
Signature: _____
Name: _____daytime phone # _____
Address: _____
City: _____ Zip _____ State _____
CA residents please add 8.25% sales tax.

S & H fees: : $5.95 for order total up to $19.99, $7.50 for order total up to $59.99, $10.00 for order total up to $99.99, $12.50 for order total up to $149.99, $16.50 for order total up to $249.99. Free shipping for orders $250+.

For fun, affordable, quality lingerie, visit
www.lingerieperfetta.com
Receive 10% off when you mention Hollywood Beauty Secrets!

HollywoodBeautySecrets
P.O.Box 10692, Marina del Rey, CA 90295
Phone: 1-877-LOUISAS (568-4727)

Loyalty Discount Order Form

Hollywood Beauty Secrets Book	13.95
Microdermabrasion Scrub	29.95
Relastyl™	56.95
Perfect RX Nite Serum	63.00
DMAE Retexturizing Crème	19.95
Age Reversal Hand Crème	16.50
Ultimate Eye Crème	39.95
Aging Eraser	47.95
Acne & Scar Crème	39.95
Astazanthin & Pycnogenol Crème	37.95
High Potency Vit. C Serum	44.95
JoinTastik	39.95
Aloe Seltzer C	26.00
Under 30-Minute Model Sculpting Workout	12.95

Method of Payment :
Sorry, no personaly checks. Cashier's Checks or Money orders only.

Visa ( ) Mastercard ( ) Amex ( ) Discover ( )

__|__|__|__|__|__|__|__|__|__|__|__|__|__|__|__

Expiration Date: _____/_____

Signature: _____

Name: _____daytime phone # _____

Address: _____

City: _____ Zip _____ State _____

CA residents please add 8.25% sales tax.

S & H fees: : $5.95 for order total up to $19.99, $7.50 for order total up to $59.99, $10.00 for order total up to $99.99, $12.50 for order total up to $149.99, $16.50 for order total up to $249.99. Free shipping for orders $250+.

For fun, affordable, quality lingerie, visit
www.lingerieperfetta.com
Receive 10% off when you mention Hollywood Beauty Secrets!

HollywoodBeautySecrets
P.O.Box 10692, Marina del Rey, CA 90295
Phone: 1-877-LOUISAS (568-4727)

Loyalty Discount Order Form

Hollywood Beauty Secrets Book	13.95
Microdermabrasion Scrub	29.95
Relastyl™	56.95
Perfect RX Nite Serum	63.00
DMAE Retexturizing Crème	19.95
Age Reversal Hand Crème	16.50
Ultimate Eye Crème	39.95
Aging Eraser	47.95
Acne & Scar Crème	39.95
Astazanthin & Pycnogenol Crème	37.95
High Potency Vit. C Serum	44.95
JoinTastik	39.95
Aloe Seltzer C	26.00
Under 30-Minute Model Sculpting Workout	12.95

Method of Payment :
Sorry, no personaly checks. Cashier's Checks or Money orders only.

Visa ( ) Mastercard ( ) Amex ( ) Discover ( )

__|__|__|__|__|__|__|__|__|__|__|__|__|__|__|__

Expiration Date: _____/_____
Signature: _____
Name: _____daytime phone # _____
Address: _____
City: _____ Zip _____ State _____

CA residents please add 8.25% sales tax.

S & H fees: : $5.95 for order total up to $19.99, $7.50 for order total up to $59.99, $10.00 for order total up to $99.99, $12.50 for order total up to $149.99, $16.50 for order total up to $249.99. Free shipping for orders $250+.

For fun, affordable, quality lingerie, visit
www.lingerieperfetta.com
Receive 10% off when you mention Hollywood Beauty Secrets!